WEIGHT OFF YOUR MIND

How to Change Your Mind About Your Body

A scientific, evidence-based approach to end binge eating, improvc body image, and facilitate weight management using hypnosis and other mind power methods

by

Dr Katie Richard

WEIGHT OFF YOUR MIND: HOW TO CHANGE YOUR MIND ABOUT YOUR BODY © Dr Katie Richard

National Library of Australia Cataloguing-in-Publication entry

Creator: Richard, Katie, author.

Title: Weight off your mind: how to change your mind about your body / Dr Katie Richard.

ISBN: 9781925497151 (paperback)
9781925497205 (eBook)

Subjects: Weight loss.
Weight loss–Psychological aspects.
Food habits–Psychological aspects.
Mind and body.

Dewey Number: 613.25

Published by **Dr Katie Richard** and InHouse Publishing
www.inhousepublishing.com.au

Dedication and Thanks

This book is dedicated to my Mama, who struggled with nicotine and alcohol addiction and a series of physical ailments, and propelled me into the pursuit of helping others with the same dilemma. Many thanks to all those who supported me in writing this book: everybody at EQ Life Design and PSI, my Angelic therapist Dianne Levick and all of my patients who provided me with the opportunity to heal. A wholehearted thanks to my awesome marketing and business mentor Angela Raspass from Ideas into Action who gave me the idea to write this book and support from my fabulous editor and friend Dr Juliette Lachemeier from The Erudite Pen and everyone at InHouse Publishing.

Table of Contents

About the Author

Dr Katie Richard, B.A., M.A., Psy.D (Clin. Psych.)

Dr Katie Richard is a clinical psychologist with over fifteen years of post-doctoral clinical experience, devoting most of her practice to helping people overcome their addictions to drugs and food. Dr Richard began her studies in 1991 in London where she trained at the Academy of Hypnotherapy and received her Certificate in Hypnotherapy & Psychotherapy. Back home in South Africa, at only nineteen years of age, she attracted patients from all over the country due to her astonishing results using only hypnotherapy. This work inspired her later doctoral project.

In 1996, she graduated from the University of Miami in Florida with a Bachelors of Arts in Psychology and Creative Writing. She then continued her formal education in San Diego at the California School of Professional Psychology at Alliant International University from which she graduated with a Master of Arts degree in Clinical Psychology in 1999. Her research in hypnosis was recognised after completing a major study at the Naval Medical Centre in San Diego. In 2001, she graduated with a Doctorate in Clinical Psychology.

She also received a Post-graduate Diploma in Social Learning Theory and Counselling from the University of Birmingham (UK) in 1998. Following her doctorate degree, she also advanced her clinical skills with training in Emotional Self-Management (ESM), training with the founders of the method (Dr Pratt & Dr Lambrou) in San Diego. She was also trained in Eye Movement Desensitisation and Reprocessing (EMDR) in 2001 and advanced her EMDR skills with the help of her supervisor Nick Cocco.

She put her clinical skills (including those in hypnosis, ESM, and EMDR) into practice when she worked in both private and public sectors in the USA, England, South Africa and Australia where she helped patients overcome mental health conditions, primarily addictions to food, alcohol, nicotine, and other drugs. In 2009, upon discovering that EMDR was successful in treating binge eating, she began working primarily with clients with food addiction, Binge Eating Disorders, and weight management problems. Combined with her fifteen years of clinical experience and her own personal experience of Binge Eating Disorder and weight management problems since age twelve, she has now forwarded her expertise in this book. She has been the primary researcher in the study of treating Binge Eating Disorder with EMDR at the University of Sydney. She presented preliminary findings at the Eating Disorder and Obesity Conference in 2015.

Dr Richard is a member of Australian Psychological Society, a registered psychologist with the Board of Psychology, a member of the Australian College of Weight Management, a member of the Professional Hypnotherapist Centre (UK), and a member of the Australasian Society on Alcohol and Other Drugs (APSAD).

Foreword

By Dr Les Blackstock

In my many years of doing cosmetic surgery including liposuction, I have been aware how much appearance impacts a person's well-being. I read an article from research at the University of New South Wales in Sydney that said that of 60,000 volunteers from all over the world, 80 percent of men and 20 percent of women who rated nearly 1,000 different female body types, the thin body type was preferred. It just goes to show that it is not only in Hollywood that men's social status is linked to the attractiveness of their wives.

Also, it is unfortunate, but the fact is, our appearance has an effect on our social status and income. Many years ago an article in the *New York Times* reported the findings of an eight-year study of 10,039 randomly selected people who were aged 16 to 24: fat women were 20 percent less likely to marry, had household incomes that were an average of $6,710 lower, and were 10 percent more likely to be living in poverty. The overweight and obese were also more likely to lose socioeconomic status. Obese men were 11 percent less likely to marry.

So, we know this is due to society's view that being overweight is unattractive. We know that 'fat' people face bullying, and when they lose weight, they get complimented. So much discrimination happens. This is not easily fixed by conventional diet and exercise programs—we know that obese and overweight people do not necessarily consume more calories than thin people.

Fortunately, help is at hand. Surgery, while it is not the only option, can be helpful. Many of my patients after surgery say, "I feel so much better about myself," and, "I am enjoying life more." They also say that liposuction surgery is able to target specific areas whereas dieting makes them lose fat from areas they don't necessarily want to lose, e.g. the breasts. So, with liposuction they can target specific areas like the thighs, abdomen, or hips.

The link between psychological well-being and change to body image is linked in both directions. Changing a person's body increases psychological well-being and the reverse is true—changing a person's psychological process improves body image and can even change body shape.

As a surgeon, I have come across people whose desire for cosmetic surgery is misplaced and the factors that drive them are actually a contra-indication to surgery. They would not be happy with the results and they are more prone to complications due to the release of negative body hormones and neuro-chemicals. I have seen evidence of these people getting psychological support and once they commit to the process, they feel so much better, even without surgery.

I know how difficult it is for people to lose weight using conventional diet and exercise programs that don't address the psychological part and don't consider the genetics of a person. We are genetically programmed to store fat. We needed it in times of plenty to save for the fasting times when we were hunter-gathers. However, in our modern society, food is everywhere, it is no wonder that we are expanding around the waist and everywhere else. For this stubborn last fat that won't shift despite exercise and diet efforts, liposuction can help.

Most people know they are not eating the right diet and that they need to exercise. What's missing is addressing the underlying psychological factors that lead to poor motivation to implement sound advice. We do not only eat because we are hungry. We eat when we are sad; we eat when are happy; we eat to please people; we eat because our mothers have told us to eat everything on the plate. The motivation to eat right, especially when it tastes so good won't come out of nowhere. Neither will you have the motivation to exercise, it'ss simply not there when you look at yourself with fat bulging over the exercise shorts. Do you really feel like showing yourself at the gym looking like that?

For this reason, I have referred many people to Dr Katie before and after liposuction and breast augmentations. Patients who were treated by Dr Katie reported stopping binge eating, no longer having cravings, being able to eat the recommended amounts of fruit and vegetables; some reported feeling more motivated to exercise. I often received reports of weight and centimetre loss but also of diminished depression. They were no longer eating to fill a void. People wanted a quick fix for major problems. While I could offer them fat loss through liposuction, I also offered them Dr Katie's help, which I knew I could rely on.

Some of the patients had other comorbid medical or personal problems that Dr Katie attended to and fought through with them. She approached each patient with sensitivity. Her passion for her calling to help people with food addiction was evident. While she wasn't able to help everyone, the one thing I saw consistently was that as long as patients had at least four sessions, binge eating ceased!

When Dr Katie initially started at our practice, she expressed feeling a bit worried she wouldn't have enough patients. But a few months later, she was working even on weekends, seeing patients back-to-back. She had patients driving all the way from as far west as Bathurst (128km away) and as far south as Caringbah (88km away) who had been referred by word-of-mouth from various patients.

I am pleased that she is now putting her expertise into this book. When Dr Katie told me she was writing a book, I was confident she would help many more people with this. So often people get misguided advice from slimming diet books and magazines and don't follow advice from specialists, even dietitians. Many people have felt disappointed in themselves in not being able to stick to a 'diet' that forbids certain foods. When Dr Katie told me about the ground-breaking research she was doing with EMDR for Binge Eating Disorder at the University of Sydney, I also realised that this is someone who has provided scientific evidence for a psychological treatment that should be used by many more practitioners.

I believe that Dr Katie's book can change people's attitude toward their bodies, their lifestyles, and their self-esteem. With Dr Katie's vast knowledge and clinical experience on this topic, it is a breath of fresh air to an area that has been polluted by people who prescribe diets and promise success. Dr Katie's approach is one that takes into account not only the physical, but also the emotional aspects involved in weight management. I believe people will finally stop blaming themselves for their failures with slimming diets with this very comprehensive reader-friendly book.

Dr Les Blackstock
Aesthetic Surgeon, Enhance Clinic, Penrith, NSW

Testimonials

Hi Dr Katie,

The EMDR technique calmed me so I was able to process feelings clearly in counselling. Previously counselling left me feeling 'swamped' by emotions but this has changed my outlook and was invaluable for my development ... I can control my portions more successfully. I eat more healthy foods, less sugar, and now exercise. A side effect of my more positive overall outlook is that I have stopped compulsive shopping! So money is less of a worry and I am more in control in that area of daily life also. I feel counselling has been a success and I am healthier, happier, and more in control because I attended sessions with you. So thanks.

R.P., NSW

Dear Dr Katie,

After seeing you for approximately 10 sessions, I just wanted to provide you with some feedback. Since seeing you for not only weight loss purposes but also to change my attitude towards the whole matter I am pleased to say I am a lot more positive towards myself these days. I wouldn't say 100% but there is definitely a difference in the way I view myself.

In relation to actually losing weight, I set a goal for myself in February this year to lose 13 kilos and I have so far lost 8 in 5 weeks. This is the first time in my entire life that I have actually been able to stick to weight loss goals set and actually stay on track. Thank you for your assistance, I just felt it important to let you know it's working!

Kind Regards, Shona Gauld, NSW

The treatment was excellent, and I found it easy to lose the weight. I feel I'm back on track, and am on the way to my goal weight. I eat a lot less sugar now, and food that is healthier. I rarely binge, and if I do I work out what the underlying problem is and I'm back on track the next day.

Thanks again, Sharon V., NSW

I have lost 4kg since treatment with you. My satisfaction with treatment with you is definitely 20 out of 10! I have had a real breakthrough in the last 2 days about finally after 50yrs as seeing food as the enemy, and my body as the war zone I am sick of it. I am choosing to see it as my friend and my eating has changed dramatically ... I am eating food that I will enjoy and healthy and mindfully eating it, no reading or watching TV. I have had no preoccupation with food and have felt full ... Now Sunday night and usually mega binge and planning on eating an enjoyable dinner including rice. I feel it is a breakthrough in how I perceive food and myself.

Pam Matthews, NSW

I found the treatment worked very quickly and I found myself more motivated to exercise and less preoccupied with food almost instantly. I have lost 17 kg!

I felt comfortable throughout the treatment—it worked after only 1 session!

S.O., NSW

Preface

How I came to develop *Weight Off Your Mind*

The idea of writing *Weight Off Your Mind* came about as I realised that I had a passion for helping people heal from overeating, obesity, and an emotional battle with their body. I had a passion because I was good at helping people heal from these—more and more, I saw results. These success stories kept happening in my practice. With my website, I also received emails from people overseas requesting my help. I wanted to reach out to more people, so I developed the 'Hyp2Hip Slimming' DVD. Through my practice, I realised some people want a bit more assistance than just the hypnosis and ESM from the DVD. In addition, I found that for some people hypnosis just didn't work and because I figured out why hypnosis didn't work, I went on a path of discovery to finding how to make hypnosis work for the resistant ones.

I have an incredible urge to get the word out there that 'diets' are not the way to cure an eating disorder. I saw too much how so many people get caught up in the diet mentality and not only fail at their weight loss attempt, but also become more and more despondent and end up hating themselves (so much more). You see: I am one of you. By that I mean: I am a 'fatty' myself, now in recovery. I not only got through Binge Eating Disorder and being overweight myself, I have also helped other people overcome their eating/weight problems.

Why I use hypnosis

When I was twelve years old I wanted to win a biathlon (a contest of running and swimming). I did not think I had any chance of winning unless I did something beyond just training daily. I searched and then came across a hypnosis book—Ursula Markham's *Hypnothink*. It inspired me and although at that stage I did not achieve my goal to win a biathlon, I became interested in hypnosis to the point that I practiced almost every day. I was able to do a trick: I was able to make a credit card stick to my forehead for several minutes even while shaking my head. I loved it!

By the time I was eighteen and ready to graduate from high school, I was eager to make a career of hypnosis. I flew to London and completed a hypnotherapy and counselling course. When I started practicing as a hypnotherapist in South Africa, I was only nineteen years old. Although I did not help everyone who came to see me, I helped many people overcome their obstacles: stuttering, smoking, poor self-confidence, cigarette addiction, etc. To me hypnosis was some kind of magic!

I believed hypnosis could do anything.

My most meaningful moment in my early career was when I had a patient in her twenties who came to me for breast cancer treatment. I had never worked with that before, but I agreed to go ahead with a hypnosis session with her because she had received positive feedback from a relative and trusted that

I would help her too. Believe it or not, I was that confident I could help her, I was disappointed the first session did not treat it!

After the second session, she phoned me to let me know she had cancelled her mastectomy as all her tumours had completely disappeared! Her doctor was shocked when he re-examined her.

I understand if you are sceptical about this cancer-cure, but to me this is just what I expected hypnosis to do. Of course, it could be argued that there were several other factors at play here i.e. her expectancy, my faith in treatment, her faith, etc. This case—although extraordinary—did not lead me onto the path of working with oncology patients as my real drive was to get the answer to alcohol and cigarette addiction because my mother struggled with these addictions for many years and I suffered as a result. Although (and perhaps because) I did not treat her, I felt compelled to help others overcome their addiction—it was therapeutic for me to eliminate other people's addictions.

I rebelled when my father and uncle pushed me to study at university, because I felt hypnosis was all I needed to know. However, I agreed to formalise my knowledge eventually. I continued to be frustrated about the sceptics about hypnotherapy at university. It was off-putting but I was determined to prove them wrong. By the time I got to Masters degree level, I found a professor Dr Jim Spira who not only supported my belief in hypnosis, he taught hypnotherapy courses. I proved my hypothesis that hypnosis works (to help people quit smoking) with my formal research project at the Naval Medical Centre in San Diego in 2001.

Despite my belief in hypnosis, I was struggling with my own crisis: I was terribly addicted to food, especially chocolate. I had been to hypnotherapists myself—not just one or two, but several, and still did not achieve my desired outcome. Neither did I succeed with the '100' diets, herbal treatments, homeopathy, appetite suppressants (Phendimetrazine), nor Tony Robbins tapes and workshops (including the Fire Walk). I (unofficially) studied nutrition and even had liposuction three times yet remained desperately unhappy with myself, my eating, and my body. I knew somehow that it was not a pill or a diet that could solve my problem, but I couldn't find the psychological solution either. My whole world revolved around finding that *one* thing that would make me stop overeating and finally get to a weight with which I was content.

I could not understand why I could treat clients and help them lose weight, but not achieve my goal weight myself. When my clients told me they were eating a whole block of chocolate driving home from the grocery store I knew exactly what that felt like. Although I never had a drug, alcohol, or cigarette addiction, I felt just like an addict when it came to food, especially chocolate. I kept thinking, *There has to be an easier way* ... and *Why can I not practice what I preach?* I do not want to be told what to eat. I ought to know it intuitively. At my heaviest I weighed 80 kg (at 5'3"/160 cm). It was driving me crazy.

Why I added ESM

After years of studying conventional psychological therapies at university, I studied Emotional Self Management (ESM) in San Diego with the founders of the method, Dr Pratt and Dr Lambrou. At the ESM workshop, I met a lady who had been abducted by the Mexican Mafia (she had been held hostage for a ransom) who had consequently been healed from her trauma by ESM. From then I knew that ESM could achieve amazing results. I also applied it to myself. It was amazing to see accelerated results with ESM added to hypnosis. I personally got temporary relief from my food addiction with the addiction of ESM. For my patients:

> ESM was a breakthrough for those who did not respond to hypnosis alone.

How eye movement desensitisation reprocessing (EMDR) revolutionised my clinical practice and changed my life

In 2001 I studied EMDR with Dr Thomas Horvath, author of *Sex, Drugs, Gambling & Chocolate.* At the time EMDR was very new, so the workshop was very basic and only 1 day long (it now is at least 4 days long). The first time I implemented EMDR, I was an intern at the San Diego Job Corps and was able to treat a young lady who had been date raped: the EMDR treatment was finalised in only one session! Because Dr Horvath was an addiction treatment expert, a past president of the Society of Addiction Psychology, he mentioned that 'EMDR could be applied to addictions' but did not go into great detail about how to do it. So, for many years, I had used it for anxiety disorders only (mostly phobias, panic attacks and PTSD).

Then in 2009 in my practice on the Gold Coast, a patient—who drove over an hour from Brisbane—was not responding to hypnosis nor ESM to relieve her addiction to junk food and chocolate. I didn't want to disappoint her, especially because she had travelled so far and was referred by someone who had achieved great results with the ESM and hypnosis. Frustrated, not knowing what to do with this desperate girl, I thought, *Maybe see if EMDR works*. Voila! It did! It was the breakthrough I needed. I researched this as I had not been taught how to apply EMDR to addictions properly when I studied EMDR in 2001. From then on, I applied it to 'food addiction' as well as those addicted to alcohol, speed, heroin, and nicotine.

EMDR seemed to resolve addiction to drugs (including nicotine) and food more effectively and faster than any other method I had been taught at university the past eight years.

It seemed that my conceptualisation as food as an addiction actually worked although the alternative explanation for it working was that Binge Eating Disorder was more like an anxiety disorder and therefore responded to EMDR (which was originally designed to treat the anxiety disorder PTSD). Once I had the treatment myself, I got results—I got to 65 kg and my eating was less compulsive, less often. Yet, the results again were temporary and somewhat laboured. There were just two more things I needed to do to make it work: firstly, I needed to find the right practitioner who understood my story and inspired me. Secondly, I needed a technique that was quick and painless. This is how I realised the power of eye movements could assist. Strange as it sounds, but eye movements used in EMDR (a scientifically supported psychological method) is also present in the breathwork, an unconventional/alternative healing method.

I also came across a method called NAET (Nambudripad Allergy Elimination Technique) that I used to get rid of my food allergies. I noticed some similarities in the method with EMDR: the method addresses that underlying emotional trauma that fuels current ailments. It all made sense to me how and why EMDR works—after all those years of practicing psychology using conventional psychological methods.

Being told what to eat, what not to eat, and to exercise, did not make sense to me. What I needed to know was *how* to do it.

Once I integrated this information, it was like something clicked and the weight dropped off me. I could eat food like a slim person. I *finally* felt the same relief that my drug addicts told me when they no longer had that tunnel vision of their drug anymore. My addiction 'food, food, food!' was no more. I could eat a piece of chocolate without having this overwhelming urge to finish off the entire block. I could share a muffin with someone. I could push the plate away—I actually felt full! I could wait for a dinner rather than feel irritated about having to wait. I could eat whatever I wanted and did not gain weight! I actually looked forward to eating salad! Eureka! With all the research I had done on nutrition and exercise, I finally was able to apply this information and then achieved my ideal body too.

My hunger did not control my life anymore.

I used EMDR on my clients and found even better and quicker results than using hypnosis and ESM. I knew I had found my purpose! I was so excited that I decided I need to get these results published in formal publications. I was advised by my professional peers to do a research degree to find scientific evidence for my findings that EMDR could be helpful in eliminating binge eating and helping people lose weight.

Doing another degree and partaking in in-depth research is not a small task, but I was so excited about this that I decided to push past the idea that it would be hard work. Despite already having a Doctorate degree, I officially enrolled as a post-graduate research student at the University of Sydney in 2013 and was conducting research on EMDR for Binge Eating Disorder. When I spoke to my supervisors, they told me this is ground-breaking and will be sought by the founder of EMDR (Dr Francine Shapiro).

I presented my preliminary research findings at the Eating Disorder and Obesity Conference in May 2015. As in my clinical practice, I found that participants had not only stopped binge eating, but had also lost weight and centimetres, and found themselves to be more motivated to exercise. That was with EMDR alone!

I am so inspired by this—I feel privileged to be able to offer something so uniquely powerful to my patients. It's a shame that the EMDR method, which has over 70,000 practitioners worldwide, is only used by just over 285 practitioners in Australia and not many (or none at all) use it specifically for (food and nicotine) addictions. I'm currently in the process of developing a training program for practitioners in Australia and other parts of the world so that many more people are able to benefit from this extraordinary method.

The results of my EMDR research were amazing and very supportive of my mission to get it across to the psychological profession that EMDR can be used to treat Binge Eating Disorder and help people lose weight. However, while ground-breaking, it was still obvious that the treatment needed improvement to apply to more people. Those who stopped binge eating but did not know what to eat, needed diet advice too; those who were inspired and motivated to exercise but didn't know which exercise to do for best results, needed exercise physiologist's advice too; those who simply did not respond to EMDR needed an alternative psychological method or an addition of medical treatment. Again, it supported my hypothesis that even the best psychological intervention I could present was incomplete or insufficient and was not applicable to everyone.

If you have been made to believe that there's something wrong with you if you can't follow this seemingly simple formula: 'eat less, exercise more', then take note—the problem is not with you. The problem is that this formula is incomplete. I believe that psychological methods have been the underdog in this whole weight management puzzle. Medical professionals—who are held in such high regard—have not been able to provide us with a satisfying answer either, and sadly not many have asked psychologists to assist in this war against obesity. When I was studying, one of my professors made us aware that she—as a psychologist—was made to feel like a second-class citizen because she was a psychologist rather than a medical professional. I have heard this sentiment more often since my studies; one of my colleagues even said that a psychiatrist told him, 'You didn't make it into medical school, so you went into psychology, huh?' In my own professional life, I have experienced being treated as inferior to a medical professional with small gestures, such as not being allotted a designated 'doctors' parking spot at the hospital, because I was not a 'real doctor'.

I am here to say that the weight management problem can be solved—not by the medical profession, not by dietitians, not by psychologists, but by acknowledging that if we all work together, we can make it happen. The only thing that is left now is to convince government regulators to stop food scientists, food manufacturers, and advertisers to fatten us up, destroying our mental and psychological health.

Introduction

'Our thoughts are traitors and make us lose the good we oft might win by fearing to attempt.'
(Shakespeare)

If you are reading this book, is it because you would like to stop binge eating or overeating, improve your body image, lose weight, and/or achieve your ideal or happy weight or all three? If this is want you want, you may notice as you continue to read this book that your belief in being able to achieve this will grow considerably. To start, identify what specifically you want (you can take a pencil and check off the ones that apply to you):

1: Have more harmonious eating patterns: no more overeating & binge eating	Check if yes
• be able to eat without losing control, even in risky situations like parties, buffets, and stressful times	
• eliminate the 'I'll start the diet on Monday' syndrome	
• be able to eat anything in moderation and abstain from binge eating forever	
• eat only when hungry rather than due to boredom, depression, anxiety, or other emotional states, or eating just to finish off what's on the plate or in the packet	

• have an appetite and hunger that is under control rather than have an existence of being controlled by an out-of-control appetite and hunger	
• be free of cravings for chocolate, carbohydrates, junk food, or food in general	
• have the ability to control food portions and speed of eating	
• improve the relationship with food by releasing anxiety about eating certain foods	
• eat any food (even cakes, chips, bread, etc.) without compulsion, guilt, or shame	
• get enough pleasure from a single bite of food instead of requiring a larger dose to feel satisfied, e.g. enjoy a small block of chocolate or one biscuit without the compulsion to eat the whole lot	
• stop feeling compelled to finish off the entire packet of biscuits, chips, etc.	
• stop self-defeating, self-destructive eating behaviour that disrupts your self-esteem	
• be drawn to eat (more) nutritious food rather than junk food	

2: Lose weight* and maintain automatically—without effort	
• lose weight without trying very hard	
• view 'diet' in a new light, see diet, not as a white-knuckle effort, but as a healthy lifestyle	
• release the obsession with food, weight, and body image issues	

* I am using the term 'lose weight' only because it is the more conventional term. If you prefer to think of this as 'releasing weight' to avoid the negative connotation of 'loss', feel free to substitute the word 'lose' with 'release'.

3: Behave and feel like a slim person	
• be in the right frame of mind to enjoy exercise	
• improve motivation to eat to improve/maintain health and energy and to meet nutritional and energy needs	
• be free of the judgment and criticism of yourself and others by eliminating the need to constantly evaluate whether you are 'good' or 'bad' depending on what you ate or how much you weigh	

4: Feel good/better about yourself	
• enjoy a positive body image, experience feeling body pride and body love and acceptance	
• enjoy improved health e.g. cholesterol, blood pressure, freedom from pain	
• enjoy better energy levels	
• feel confident (and become a better role model for children and others)	
• be able to cope with stressors by improved coping skills and better social support rather than by eating	
• enjoy improved mood and general wellbeing	
• have improved overall appearance (improve hair, nails, skin)	

So, is all of this possible or it is just a dream? As you read through *Weight Off Your Mind*, wondering how you can achieve what you want, and while you are letting go of old limiting beliefs, you will discover exactly what magic can happen. Your weight, your body, and your eating can all change for the better.

Other slimming books and programs have gone by the assumption that weight loss and maintenance is simply a one-size fits all calorie-in, calorie-out formula. That is the reason so many of them fail. *Weight Off Your Mind* is different.

The 4 reasons *Weight Off Your Mind* could help you normalise your eating and achieve and maintain your happy weight/shape

Reason #1: The barriers to achieve success with hypnosis are addressed

Hypnosis can work and does work, but there are so many other factors that may need to be addressed in order for hypnosis to work. Having originally trained as a hypnotherapist and achieving success with hypnosis, I am definitely a big supporter of using hypnosis for weight management. However, as you will read in the chapter on hypnosis, not much scientific literature supports the use of hypnosis, especially as a stand-alone method for Binge Eating Disorder and weight management problems. The fact that hypnotherapy does not have much scientific evidence to support its efficacy isn't because it's not effective though. Although the well-known psychologist Sigmund Freud used hypnosis, it never gained enough ground and hence was never regarded as an evidence-based psychological method.

Sadly, because of this, there are many hypnotherapists out there who may not be properly trained. Many hypnotherapists practice hypnotherapy after undergoing a weekend training workshop. Hypnosis books also consequently fail to provide the extraordinary outcomes that hypnosis is capable of. Neither are hypnotherapists screened—as other health professionals—to ensure that they are even suitable to practice in this profession. Some practitioners may also lack basic psychological knowledge to actually practice hypnotherapy. Therefore, the quality of hypnotherapy provided is poor. As you will discover when you read the hypnosis chapter, there is so much more to hypnosis than going into trance and listening to a standardised hypnosis script.

In addition, when hypnosis is researched in a proper scientific manner, it is either the method or the therapists themselves that provide disappointing results. So, we rely on case studies that end up being more of a 'he said, she said' piece of evidence. Some hypnotherapists advertising on the internet claim to get fabulous results immediately. I too can provide multiple reports of people who have quit binge eating and lost weight with my hypnosis sessions. However, the truth is, hypnosis (especially as a stand-alone method) does not always work and is not applicable or appropriate for everyone. If you've ever been to a hypnotherapy session, you may have found that it either doesn't work at all or works temporarily or only partially. If you've ever read a hypnosis book or used a hypnosis CD, you may have not succeeded at all.

This is how *Weight Off Your Mind* is different. It's not a book about weight loss with hypnosis only—not because hypnosis doesn't work. It's not a book about weight loss with hypnosis only because there are potentially many other factors that need to be considered in order to make hypnosis most effective. *Weight Off Your Mind* is a book about how to make hypnosis work for you because in my many years of experience with weight management, hypnosis is the easiest way to do it. The good news is: I will let you into the secrets!

Whereas other slimming books or CDs will promise that hypnosis will help you achieve your weight management goals, the truth is: overcoming weight/eating/body image problems with hypnosis alone is the exception rather than the rule. I myself struggled with the idea that hypnosis alone is insufficient. My personal experience with hypnosis (in which I failed to achieve weight loss with it), as well as years of clinical practice, has confirmed that sadly, hypnosis by itself may not work.

Weight Off Your Mind differs in at least two ways to other slimming books and other hypnosis books. Firstly, *Weight Off Your Mind* has subliminal (hypnotic) suggestions throughout—this means that as you are reading it, you will already start programming yourself to achieve your happy weight and harmonise your eating patterns. You may or may not notice this, but you will absorb suggestions to lose weight, quit binge eating, quit overeating and notice some other surprising pleasant side-effects. If you wonder how all of this works and what the outcome will be, keep reading. You will discover the magic power of hypnosis as you read.

Secondly, *Weight Off Your Mind* was written after extensive experience and trial and error over many years with thousands of case studies (since 1991), as well as extensive review of the scientific literature on weight management. The outcome of all of this combined was that hypnosis can work but only if it's used as part of a multi-pronged approach.

The fact that weight management needs to be tackled from a wholistic approach was also clear from a presentation I attended at the Eating Disorder and Obesity Conference in Queensland in May 2014. Psychologist and dietitian Dr Anita Cochrane outlined her research she conducted at the Queensland University of Technology in which she investigated the need for a multi-component, multi-disciplinary approach to manage problematic eating and obesity. She confirmed that physicians alone do not have the answer; dietitians alone do not have the answer; exercise physiologists alone do not have the answer; psychologists alone do not have the answer. But by combining diet, exercise, psychological, and medical components, the weight problem can be tackled.[1]

Even my former high school classmate, a dietitian for Run/Walk for Life for the past 15 years and a contestant in the ultra-marathon Comrades, asked me to help her with her binge eating and weight problem. Clearly all the knowledge in nutrition and all that exercise did not help her solve her own weight problem. A psychological (or possibly medical) intervention or change in exercise type may have been more successful. It's the same reason even well-known TV personality personal trainers with weight loss shows don't just make people exercise. They tell them to change their diet and say things to motivate them to implement these changes. As you know, these personal trainers are not experts in diet nor psychological intervention, but they apply all these components to get results. That's the reason I too am applying mind methods as well as an exercise and diet component.

The idea of an integrated approach is not unique to weight management and problematic eating. Since 1998 when I was first engaged in treating people with drug and alcohol addictions, we always spoke about an 'integrated' approach. Still years later, when I worked at Queensland Health hospital, we were given a clinical guideline that advised us to apply this integrated approach. We were clinicians expected not to treat the drug addiction in isolation of other factors; it was assumed that we would take care of the issues connected with the addiction: mental health problems, homelessness, medical issues, educational problems, etc. So, why not treat Binge Eating Disorder and weight management problems with an integrated approach, when it's clearly linked to psychological, medical, and/or social problems?

What is clear from decades of research in the eating disorder and obesity literature is that weight and eating problems need to be tackled from a multi-component approach that includes diet, exercise, and behavioural counselling.[2]

It is for this reason that *Weight Off Your Mind* has a chapter on diet, 'What to eat to slim down'; one chapter on exercise, 'How the new science in exercise can boost your weight loss'; and all the other chapters are psychological methods that will remove the barriers to succeeding with hypnosis. You will also be pleased to know that it has one additional factor that is part of that multi-component approach that 99 percent of other slimming books neglect—an entire chapter on how to overcome potential medical/physical barriers with the chapter entitled 'Dr to the rescue'. I believe it's irresponsible for medical doctors (who are not usually specificially trained in weight management) to publish slimming books unless the psychological, diet and exercise components are mentioned, but I do believe GPs can provide valuable insights into potential medical obstacles. Therefore, you may be happy to know that your GP can be of great assistance.

> Attempting to fix your Binge Eating Disorder by going on another fad diet is not the solution; in fact, going on another 'diet' without psychological support is likely to worsen it

Reason #2: Hypnosis is potentiated with other psychological methods

As mentioned above, hypnosis is a very powerful method that can help you achieve your weight management goal as it makes eating in moderation and exercising regularly easy. As you may have read in the preface, as magic as hypnosis is, by itself hypnosis may be insufficient. This is partly, as mentioned above, that hypnosis may be ineffective if administered by untrained, inexperienced practitioners who may just read a standard hypnosis script while you're in a trance state.

However, hypnosis may also not be sufficient because it may not be able to address major obstacles including poor self-esteem, poor self-efficacy, resentment, poor coping skills, insufficient stress management skills, and other mental health problems (especially mood and anxiety disorders). This is how *Weight Off Your Mind* differs from other slimming books. Research after research has shown how complex weight/eating issues are. Consequently, treatment needs to correspond to its complexity. I see it as the equivalent of someone walking to the doctors to get treatment for a burst appendix. The level of care needed to treat a more complex problem has to match the complexity of the presenting symptoms. Just as you need to be hospitalised (not just given tablets by a GP) for a burst appendix, so too do you need a more multi-faceted treatment for disordered eating and a weight problem. A diet alone is grossly insufficient. You need to be given the right information as well as the necessary treatment, not just a diet and exercise program by people who aren't sufficiently qualified. From my clinical experience, I have seen how attempting to address weight management/eating issues without addressing self-esteem, for example, is bound to lead to failure. The research too shows that repeatedly failing on diet program leads to diminished self-esteem.[3] If you have poor self-esteem and feel ineffective, you are less likely to feel motivated to try again.[4]

In addition, the scientific literature is full of evidence showing how the presence of depression decreases the chance of success in weight loss programs.[4] A systematic review and analysis of 112,708 participants in the journal *Obesity Review* found that adults with reported childhood abuse were significantly more likely to be obese and yet other slimming books never address trauma and resentment.[5] *Weight Off Your Mind* will assist you in overcoming the trauma with psychological methods including EMDR and a very powerful chapter on harnessing the power of forgiveness.

I felt that the inclusion of psychological methods was so crucial too, it was evident—not only from my clinical practice but also from the literature—that it's virtually impossible not to regain weight if you continue to eat in response to negative emotions and stress.[6] A study published in the *American Journal of Clinical Nutrition* found key differences between 44 relapsers and 30 maintainers: 95 percent of maintainers confronted problems directly (compared to 10 percent of relapsers) and used personally developed strategies to help themselves.[7]

Similar findings were reported in an article entitled 'Who succeeds in maintaining weight loss?' in the journal *Obesity Reviews*.[8] Researchers *found that* successful weight maintenance (defined as maintaining weight loss for at least 6 months) is associated with more initial weight loss, achieving a self-determined goal weight, a physically active lifestyle, a regular meal rhythm including eating healthily and eating breakfast, absence of loss of control of over eating, and self-monitoring of behaviours. Weight maintenance was linked to having a strong motivation to lose weight, a supportive social network, better coping strategies, especially an ability to cope with stressors, high self-efficacy, assuming responsibility in life, and more psychological strength and stability.

Weight regain was associated with a history of weight cycling, disinhibited eating, binge eating, more hunger, eating in response to negative emotions and stress, and more passive reactions to problems.[9]

That's the reason there's a whole chapter on how to build self-efficacy, a social support network, eliminate binge eating/comfort eating, stress management, and various ways to cope with unpleasant emotions and problems.

Reason #3: Everything is backed up by solid scientific evidence

Unlike conventional slimming books that base their entire theory on a single study, this book is based on hundreds of case studies, as well as hundreds of studies that have been published in recognised professional journals. You may have noticed that the pages of references (sources) at the end of this book. It's not just a single page. If you were to look at books written on a 'good fat' diet, the author may quote one, or at the most two, scientific studies or case studies. For example, The Fatburner Diet provides evidence that it works based on only 14 volunteers! It goes on to recommend avoiding sugar, including chocolate, when there is mountains of evidence that sugar does not 'make you fat', as well as realms of scientific evidence that forbidding a certain food can actually make your Binge Eating Disorder worse.

I am not suggesting that the author is basing his 'good fat' theory on no evidence at all. I believe he is being genuine when he reports cases of success with this diet. However, if you were told that 140 participants who took part in a scientifically conducted study with rigorous research methodology on a particularly weight management method showing an average weight loss of 10kg in 3 months, would you trust that? Or would you trust an author who quotes that 14 volunteers reported to a magazine that they had lost an average of 10kg in 3 months? I believe that saying any diet or pill or potion works based on a few case studies is irresponsible. The reason that major pharmaceutical companies are able to sell their medication is that in medical studies the product is tested on thousands of people before it is marketed. It's not unusual for it to be tested on at least 1,000 people in phase one of a human trial. How any slimming program gets sold with only a few case studies or one or two clinical trials can be explained only by our vulnerability and desperation, fuelled by our trust and belief in the authors, or manipulation by clever marketing tactics.

You can rest assured that *Weight Off Your Mind* is based not only on my personal experience but also on hundreds of my own case studies over my 15 years in clinical practice, hundreds of research articles in scientific journals, as well as the study I conducted at the University of Sydney. The glossary of terms at the back will explain some research terms if you are unclear about terms like 'randomised controlled trial'.

> 'The waist is a terrible thing to mind. The mind is a terrible thing to waste.' *(Anonymous)*

Reason #4: Weight loss and maintenance becomes an easy, effortless process

You may be familiar or unsurprised by the statistics of rate of failure with weight loss maintenance. In other words, you're not alone if you haven't succeeded yet. According to a report in the *Annual Review of Nutrition* 80 percent of people are unable to maintain a weight loss of at least 10 percent for more than a year.[9] In contrast, researchers at the University of Kansas Medical Centre found that of 179 participants, 76.5 percent had successfully maintained their weight loss of at least 5 percent. One of their conclusions was that maintainers were those who were able to reduce the level of perceived effort required for long-term weight control.[10]

In other words, if you are just 'white-knuckling' a diet, holding your breath until you can eat what you want, you are less likely to succeed. Another study of 931 participants, published in *Obesity Research* echoed this finding.[1] It makes sense: if you find it easy to eat in moderation and exercise on a regular basis, you will continue with it. But how to make it effortless? If this appears like a pipe dream to you, rest assured. You will may be surprised how much hypnosis (and the other strategies outlined that in *Weight Off Your Mind* that potentiate hypnosis) make it easier for you.

You will also discover that while preventing weight regain after weight loss is one of the greatest challenges for most people, weight maintenance is actually easier than weight loss.[12] In fact, maintenance for some people gets easier over time and the chance of relapse after two years is unlikely.[13]

The research says that dietary/lifestyle programs are suitable for people who want to lose up to 5kg or for those with a BMI 25.0–29.9kg/m2 with two or more risk factors; that pharmacological therapy (Orlistat, Topiramate or appetite suppressants, e.g. Duramine) are for those who want to lose up to 10kg or those with a BMI of 30–39 kg/m2 or have failed with diet and exercise program; and bariatric surgery is suitable for those seeking a weight loss of 25–75kg or for those with a BMI of 40 kg/m2 or more and those who have comorbid conditions (i.e. health problems).[14,15] Yet, there is vast amount of evidence that even those who have undergone bariatric surgery require dietary/lifestyle treatment—in other words, bariatric surgery does not mean you don't also have to change your eating and (lack of) exercise habit. Sadly, although the evidence for pharmacological is good in the short-term, provided the negative side effects are minimal, tablets are never the long term solution nor a cure.

Weight Off Your Mind is designed to provide you with the tools to eliminate the root causes of your weight/eating problems. It's designed for you if you prefer the easy and sure way out of your 'food addiction'. Whether you need to lose 5kg or 30kg or have undergone bariatric surgery, I believe this book will help you. I wish you all the best! When you have read Weight Off Your Mind, please do me a favour: send me your feedback!

Part I

How to Make Hypnosis Work by Removing Physical/Medical Barriers

Chapter 1: **Body Check**

'I've been on a constant diet for the last 2 decades. I've lost a total of 789 pounds. By all accounts, I should be hanging off a charm bracelet.'
(Erma Bombeck)

Step 1 to prepare your body for your slimming journey is all about investigating if any physical/medical barriers are in the way of your success. In my clinical practice, it's actually very rare for me not to refer a patient to a GP for a medical check-up. There are several reasons for this:

- To identify if there's a medical/physical condition that is affecting your weight or appetite
- To assess whether medication (if you're on any) is affecting your weight/appetite
- To get biofeedback on your before and after health status, which can serve as an incentive to keep going with a healthy lifestyle

Dr to the Rescue #1: Do I Have a Medical Condition That Affects My Weight/Appetite?

Thyroid problems: It's perhaps because thyroid disorders are so rarely a cause of a weight problem that it is often missed. Indeed, thyroid problems are present in only about 10 percent of people.[1] In all of my years in clinical practice with overweight and obese people who have came to me for help to lose weight, I suspected and referred only a few patients to assess the presence of a thyroid problem. However, in each case, getting a confirmation by a thyroid test was the key to opening the door to the patient's weight loss journey.

I had a patient in her late twenties who was referred by her GP for 'depression' due to having had a miscarriage. Unfortunately, he did not think to test her for anything, referred her to me right away, and gave her a prescription for anti-depressants. During my assessment with her I discovered that she felt not only depressed (because of the miscarriage, but also because of weight problems), but also fatigued, had frequent headaches, a poor sex drive and a hoarse voice. I advised her to go to a GP to get physical conditions ruled out, suggesting 'perhaps the GP wants to do a thyroid test'. She agreed to go to a GP who tested for several things including thyroid function. She was so glad she did, because it confirmed that she did indeed have hypothyroidism. Not only was she then treated for hypothyroidism, she also had an explanation for her miscarriage as well as her depression. Of course, because she was then correctly treated, she was also then able to lose weight and exercise due to increased energy.

Another one of my patients had post-partum thyroid problems, but had she not checked this out she would have continued to blame her fatigue, weight problems, and consequent lack of progress with my sessions on the baby! For further information read the book *Your Thyroid Problems Solved* (Dr Sandra Cabot). Or, go to any of the following websites:

www.aace.com/files/hypothyroidism_guidelines.pdf
www.betterhealth.vic.gov.au
www.btf-thyroid.org
www.thyroid.about.com
www.thyroidmanager.org
www.thyroid.org.au

Insulin problems: Whereas insulinoma, hyperinsulinemia, and congenital hyperinsulinism are rare disorders, Insulin Resistance, also known as Metabolic Syndrome or Syndrome X, is present in about 5 million Australians. According to research published in the journal *Metabolism*, 'hyperinsulinemia results in increased hunger, heightened palatability of sucrose or sweetness, and greater food intake.'[2] The Australian Diabetes, Obesity and Lifestyle study (AusDiab) in 2000 found that 19 percent of Australians aged twenty-five years and over met the criteria for the metabolic syndrome diagnosis.[3] Insulin problems too, unfortunately, are often missed as people attribute their symptoms to a stressful lifestyle.

But because my assessment always includes a physical check-up, I've been able to catch this in several people and thus have been able to help eliminate this obstacle. I remember one patient who came to me as she struggled to lose weight, had food cravings, and felt hungry all the time. She was no different from most of my other patients. Like many other patients, she also complained about feeling anxious, restless, fatigued, sleepy, having trouble concentrating, and having frequent headaches. As a psychologist, it would have been easy to attribute all of these symptoms to a psychological disorder, e.g. a major depressive disorder. Fortunately, I sent her back to her GP who tested her blood pressure, cholesterol, and fasting glucose. She was diagnosed and treated hormonally. Thanks to this diagnosis and consequent treatment, she no longer had her body going against her mind in her weight loss journey. I've had other people who had similar symptoms and were diagnosed with Polycystic Ovarian Syndrome (Stein-Levanthal Syndrome).

Testosterone problems: I had another patient who presented with weight problems who was grateful I checked out his physical condition first. My assessment revealed that—apart from weight problems - he felt fatigued, depressed, had poor sex drive, felt restless, irritable and had restless sleep. All these symptoms could've led me to the conclusion that these were just symptoms of depression, but I thought I would just make sure first if there was a physical condition at the root of this. Fortunately, sending him to his GP made all the difference as he was diagnosed with testosterone deficiency. Not only did testosterone treatment help him lose weight, imagine the surprise his wife got when his sex drive and sexual functioning improved!

Research on treating testosterone deficiency with testosterone treatment, presented at the 19th European Congress on Obesity in France, revealed that not only did participants (who were older, overweight men) show improvements in blood pressure, blood glucose, LDL (bad) cholesterol, and erectile function, they also lost more than 30 pounds on average over the course of the study! Thus, imagine if you have this problem and keep wondering why hypnosis is not working. Thus, if you're a man, it would be a great idea to get your testosterone levels checked.

Nutrient deficiencies: Over the many years of working with patients with eating disorders, I can see what is meant by the phrase 'overfed but undernourished'. If you're a binge eater and struggle to choose to eat fruits and vegetables in favour of ice cream, chocolate, cakes, chips, biscuits, etc., or are vegetarian, it's even more likely that you may have a nutritional deficiency. Of course, you know that not only does the amount of food but also the type of food affect your appetite and hence weight, but you may not realise that a simple nutritional remedy can significantly assist in stopping the depressing binge eating/overeating process.

It's a fairly typical presentation—like a patient who attended treatment with me saying her appetite was out of control, food cravings galore, poor motivation to exercise, etc. She was vegetarian, so when I sent her off to the GP, I specifically wanted her to be tested for vitamin B12, iron, and vitamin D. It was no surprise to me, but when she was diagnosed with vitamin B12 deficiency and was given supplementation, her energy improved instantly, giving her enough energy to exercise every day. All that and we hadn't even started out with hypnosis yet.

I had another patient who consulted me due to failure with bariatric surgery. She mentioned having to drink loads of coffee to boost her energy levels and attributed her weight gain to all the sugar she added to her coffee. She said she didn't want to exercise as her muscles were already sore. After sending her for blood tests, she was found to be suffering with iron-deficiency anaemia. After supplementing with iron for a few weeks, her fatigue alleviated, she stopped drinking so much coffee (and hence also had less sugar), and her appetite was more in control. With a blood test that confirmed this physical obstacle to her weight management journey, she didn't even need hypnosis!

I've also had a few patients who found out they were coeliac (gluten intolerant) and thus were unable to absorb iron. Thus after going to a GP, they not only found out they needed to avoid bread, pasta, and other gluten products, they also supplemented with iron which then actually absorbed. This is the difference between just going to get supplements yourself without consultation versus finding out what's actually causing the deficiency in the first place.

Another patient, who at sixty-two years of age complained that she ought to have her weight under control by now, told me that she attributed her obesity to lack of exercise 'which is strange because my bones and muscles are sore even without exercise'. She stated she didn't like exercising anyway as it was too hot outside. I sent her off to the GP, which revealed she actually had vitamin D deficiency! I've had many other people with the same problem—mostly those who are vegan, have had a gastric bypass, or don't spend a great deal of time out in the sunshine. All of them found that once the supplemented with vitamin D (typically around 1,000 iu), they not only felt better, the weight also dropped off fairly quickly.

According to the literature, vitamin D deficiency is actually associated with obesity—whether it's a cause or a result is still in debate. However, so far, a systematic review and meta-analysis of 23 studies published in the journal *Obesity Review* confirmed that the prevalence of vitamin D deficiency was 35 percent higher in obese subjects compared to the non-obese group and 24 percent higher than in the overweight group.[5] A study published in the *British Journal of Nutrition* reported an investigation on the effect of vitamin D supplementation on weight loss. They found that participants with adequate vitamin D levels responded better to low calorie diets (lost more body fat) than those with inadequate vitamin

D.[6] Another study of 77 people even found that supplementation of vitamin D3 (25 ug) alone (without diet) was effective in reducing body fat—in fact, it lead to 2.7kg reduction in 12 weeks.[7]

In fact, researchers have actually found that vitamin D actually regulates fat cells. More specifically, they discovered that not only are obese people more at risk of vitamin D deficiency but they are also more likely to suffer insulin and metabolism problems. They therefore recommend vitamin D supplementation with exercise and calorie restriction.[8] There is also evidence that vitamin D supplementation may assist people regulate their insulin levels.

Other than vitamin B12, iron and vitamin D, there are many other nutrients that may play a role in your weight management struggle. For example, data from six observational studies and three controlled trials have confirmed that calcium (mostly around 1500 mg per day) is associated with weight loss.[9] Rather than just go out and get supplements, I would urge you to go to a GP first to get a blood test or further investigation to see which physical causes are exactly at the root of your problem. If your GP is unable to advise on supplementation, a consultation with a nutritionist may be useful to ensure you're taking the correct dose for sufficient amount of time.

Apart from hypothyroidism, insulin problems, testosterone deficiency and nutrient deficiencies, your GP may be able to investigate other causes for your weight/eating problems. One option is to simply ask your GP 'could there be a medical explanation and hence a solution?' Alternatively, the next few chapters may be able to provide further insights into what may be the problem e.g. if your periods are irregular and you have other pre-menstrual symptoms, it may be worth mentioning this to your GP who could do a hormone test. A had a patient who I diagnosed with Premenstrual Dysphoric Disorder (typically referred to as 'PMS' and consequently sent to the GP for hormone testing. Her oestrogen was only slightly abnormal, so her GP advised her to start the Pill, multi-vitamins with extra iron and also Prozac (which is a more common prescription for PMS in the USA). Within 3 months, she no longer met criteria for the diagnosis and the weight came off without a struggle.

Dr to the Rescue #2: Am I Taking Medication That is Contributing to My Weight/Appetite Gain?

Whereas I would caution against not taking a prescribed medication just because of risk of weight/fat gain and increased appetite, be aware that some medication could be hindering you. Do not go against medical advice. However, a second opinion about a medication may save you from the unwanted side-effects, especially if they include increased appetite and/or weight gain. The following is a list of potential culprits:

Corticosteroids: I've had several people over the years come to me for weight problems following use of corticosteroids (e.g. prednisone) for conditions such as arthritis. Most of them had an increased appetite, water retention, and had gained weight (about 7–10 percent) and had fat, particularly around the abdomen. When they made their GP aware that they would like to switch to a different anti-inflammatory, they were usually given aspirin or similar painkiller. If you are prescribed steroids, be sure to discuss the risk of increased appetite, weight and fat with your prescriber.

Contraceptives: I've had many women complaining of weight gain particularly with Implanon, although a recent Cochrane review of 49 trials that included 85 weight change comparisons for 52 distinct contraceptive pairs (or placebos) showed that in general, the Pill does not lead to weight change.[10] If you've noticed an increase in appetite or weight since commencing contraceptives, talk to your GP about alternatives.

Diabetes medication (e.g. sulfonylureas, diabenese): I've had several patients complain that these stimulate hunger. Other diabetes medication, e.g. thiazolidinediones (TZDs), may cause some people to retain water/salt. If you've found that you've gained weight since starting your diabetes medication, talk to your GP. He or she may be able to prescribe alternatives including biguanides and Dpp-4 inhibitors. I had a patient who started the diabetes medication Metformin and actually lost 5kg! For further information on Metformin and other weight loss medications, look out for my book *Hyp2Hip Slimming*.

Allergy medications (Allegra, Diphenhydramine): I've heard only from friends and a few patients that anti-histamines can increase appetite, but I haven't found much scientific evidence of this. However, if you are taking anti-histamines and have noticed an increased appetite, talk to your GP about alternatives. Although not scientifically-based, the allergy elimination treatment NAET may be an alternative option.

Blood pressure medications: Some patients come to me at a stage when their weight has already caused health problems only to be given medication that makes their appetite/weight even worse. Several people who have come to me for weight problems have reported increased weight problems after taking beta blockers—apparently, they not only decrease metabolism, they also limit heartbeat, thus preventing you from exercising at full capacity. Talk to your GP about a possible alternative like Angiotension.

Anti-psychotics and mood stabilisers: All anti-psychotics (e.g. Depakote, Lithium, Zyprexa, Thorazine, etc.) have the potential to lead to weight gain.[11] Alternatives may be difficult to find but discuss possible options with your psychiatrist.

Anti-depressants: Some anti-depressants are notorious for weight gain. In many years in practice with patients who took anti-depressants, the main culprits appear to be Endep, Imipramine, Clomipramine, Nortriptyline, Avanza, Paxil/Arapax, Remeron, and Reboxetine. On the other hand, I've seen people on Prozac (Fluoxetine) and Wellbutrin (Zyban/bupropion) actually lose weight. Discuss options with your GP if you are currently on an anti-depressant that's making you gain weight or if you are planning to start an anti-depressant.

Dr to the Rescue #3: How Can I Get Proof That My Change of Lifestyle is Affecting Me?

I had a patient who came to me after successfully quitting smoking and said, 'I've actually considered taking it up again as I don't feel any better.' Of course, after I urged her to get a check-up from the GP, she reported that her blood pressure and cholesterol had actually improved since quitting. Had she not done this, she may have reverted back to the habit of smoking. I have found a similar thing with my weight management patients.

Imagine eating fewer sweets, smaller portions, more vegetables, and losing 5kg but not feeling other expected benefits. I've only discovered recently how valuable it is to have patients get a before and after health check (as well as a photo) with their GP based on a few patients reporting having improved blood pressure, cholesterol (and hence all sorts of reductions in risk of heart disease) as well as of course, reduced risk of diabetes. One patient in particular reported improved test results on her LFT (liver function test) which motivated her to continue with her healthier diet.

Prepare your body for weight management by asking your GP to:

- ✓ test your TSH (thyroid) and fasting glucose (insulin),
- ✓ (if you're male), test testosterone
- ✓ test your vitamin D, iron and vitamin B12 levels, particularly if you restrict your diet
- ✓ check out whether your medication is causing you weight management problems
- ✓ to maintain motivation to stay on a healthy diet, ask your GP to check your blood pressure, cholesterol and do a Liver Function Test (LFT)

Part II

How to Make Hypnosis Work by Removing Life Barriers

Chapter 2: **Believe It or Not**

'Most of the things worth doing in the world had been declared impossible before they were done.'
(Supreme Court Justice Louis D. Brandeis)

If someone were to tell you that you could lose all the weight you want to and easily maintain your ideal weight, achieve control over your eating and have a happy body image, would you believe it? My guess—since you are reading this book now—is that there's a part of you that believes this is possible, but another part that is a bit sceptical. The latter part is understandable if you are like so many who have gone through countless efforts to slim down and/or regulate your eating and have been met with repeated failures. The fact is: without believing that you can achieve your goals, you are unlikely to achieve your goals. In other words, believing that you can achieve them is a very important factor. Belief in yourself—having self-efficacy—is one of the most crucial aspects in achieving your weight management goal. The second part of success is believing in the way you are going about achieving this goal. This is the reason this belief chapter is in the beginning chapters of *Weight Off Your*

Mind. When you read the hypnosis chapter, you will again be reminded that it is the belief in hypnosis as well as in yourself that will enable the hypnosis to work.

Taking the Journey From Self-Doubt to Confidence

If you have any doubt that you will succeed, start by taking the steps now to full belief. It's the most important transformational trip you need to take to succeed in your weight management goal. This is because one of the key differences between those who succeed and those who do not is believing it will happen. Believing in yourself, known as having high 'self-efficacy' means that you have the confidence or the belief in your ability to succeed in something. A study published in the journal *Nutrition Research* found that participants who had higher total self-efficacy, and self-efficacy to resist eating when food was available, were able to lose more weight (3.6–7.1kg) than those low on self-efficacy.[1] Thus, instead of dwelling in despair that you have tried and tried again without success, you can revel in the following facts:

- repeated attempts to change lead to success[2]
- provided you are hopeful, when you do fail at something, you are more likely to revise your expectancies and generate more effective routes to your goals[3]
- the more weight loss attempts you have had, the greater likelihood of success[4]

The fact is: weight loss and relief from problematic eating and poor body image is achievable and realistic. If you look at the scientific literature on the success rates of smokers quitting with the help of nicotine therapy, you will see relapse rates of about 70–80 percent[5]—in other words, a success rate of 20–30 percent too. Research has also found that smokers have 5–7 serious quit attempts before quitting for good.[6] Yet, smokers are not told 'don't bother attempting to quit smoking—it doesn't work'. So why should we bingers/overeaters give up because our third or fifth attempt hasn't worked yet? Especially when were are given the wrong information about how to do it?

How to Build Your Self-Efficacy Muscle

The good news is that self-efficacy is not a stable personality trait. Rather, you can enrich your self-efficacy, just like you can learn a skill like riding a bicycle. Researchers at the University of Manchester have confirmed, for example, that boosting participants' self-efficacy dealing with temptations to eat, improved their likelihood of success with weight loss.[7] This makes sense. If you are confident that you can resist, you will.

So, how is self-efficacy improved? One way is to look at your past successes (in any area) which builds a mindset of success: 'I've succeeded in something else that I hadn't tried before, so I can succeed in this (weight loss/eating) goal too.' For example, imagine having to cook a three course meal for six people for the first time. How would you believe you could do it? Do you base this belief on the fact that you have done something similar before, e.g. you have cooked a two course meal for two people before?

Another way to enhance your self-efficacy is to look at how someone else is succeeding and emulate that. For example, if you wanted to succeed in a new business, do you think it would help if you were to talk to business mentors who have succeeded in business already? It's the same reason that an apprentice learns from his mentor; a student learns from a professor; an Alcoholics Anonymous member learns to stay sober with the help of a 'sponsor' (a person who has had long term sobriety). The chapter on social support will explain this part in more detail. However, the point to keep in mind here is: if all of those people can do it, so can you! Look at all these successful maintainers in the National Weight Control Registry:

If they can do it, you can do it too

The National Weight Control Registry (NWCR) is an ongoing registry of individuals (over 10,000) who have been successful at losing and maintaining a minimum of 13.6kg for at least 1 year. 80 percent of people in the registry are women and 20 percent are men. The 'average' woman in the NWCR is 45 years of age and currently weighs 145lbs (~66kg), while the average man is forty-nine years of age and currently weighs 190lbs (~86kg). Registry members have lost an average of 66lbs (~30kg) and kept it off for 5.5 years. Weight losses have ranged from 30lbs (~14kg) to 300 lbs (~136kg). Years of maintenance ranged from 1 year to 66 years! Some have lost the weight rapidly, while others have lost weight very slowly—over as many as 14 years. 45 percent reported losing the weight entirely on their own (usually diet and physical activity) rather than through a program. 42 percent found maintenance easier than weight loss. (Details derived from: www.nwcr.ws)

A third way to boost your self-efficacy is to change the way you think. Obviously, this is the core of *Weight Off Your Mind* and as you read through, you will gain more mastery of your skill to train your mind to think slim. To start out with, here's a quick trick to change your mind about yourself in regards to self-efficacy: we call it 'reframing'. Reframing means you view things from another perspective—think of a picture you place in a different frame to give it a fresh appeal. The reason it's helpful to reframe in self-efficacy is that you can move past seeing what you have done so far as 'failures'. By looking at your previous efforts to do anything, including trying to lose weight or change your eating, start an exercise regime as practice runs rather than as 'failures', you can increase your self-efficacy.

So, your belief in being able to change can be improved by you continually building on your past successes, watching and emulating other successful people, and changing the way to think. It's one step up from just thinking positively. In fact, if you think just like the masses, you will be just like everyone else. So, it's thinking positively but also thinking outside the box. If you have watched a popular weight loss show on TV, you will have seen, for example, that weight loss is about being screamed at by a personal trainer and being told you cannot eat your favourite foods. Most slimming books have a similar message. But does that work? Evidently for some, but not for the majority, particularly the ones who don't even commence on a change of diet and exercise program. But if you think outside the box, you may find that you can easily dismiss what conventional slimming programs have told you. A friend of mine once told me about a delicatessen shop that stocks German Christmas baked goods but added, 'But you can't eat those, can you?' He asked this question because he assumed that because I was 'watching my weight' that I couldn't eat those delicious German bakery goods. Convention says 'don't eat sweets', but why stick with this convention when you can break it and still maintain a slim figure?

Continuing with the idea that your slimming journey may require you to think outside the conventional and you are willing to try something less 'normal', then you may welcome the thought of engaging the forces around you—whether you are a spiritual person or not—to achieve something extraordinary. If you are open-minded but still want scientifically-based extra support, you can use this resource. If you prefer to stick to the conventional, skip the next section on how you can harness the power of a higher power to assist you in your weight management goal.

Ask and You Shall Receive

This section is for you if you are willing to ask a higher power or God to assist you. Thus, it will apply if you feel that you need more than what conventional methods can offer you. If you have ever heard of people praying for something and having their prayers answered, this section will provide you with the tools to help you use the power of prayer to get and stay slim. Using prayer, a faith in God, or a higher power, I have seen miracles in people—even in people who didn't consider themselves to be religious or god-fearing— recover from a variety of illnesses!

As I mentioned in the preface, I saw with my own eyes a patient healing from breast cancer using faith and my hypnosis session. Miraculously, all eight tumours in her breast disappeared after only one therapy session—she had to actually cancel her mastectomy surgery as the scans could no longer detect the tumours! Incredible, yet even scientific research has proven how powerful prayer can be. For example, a study headed by cardiac researcher Dr Harris found the positive effects of intercessory prayer in cardiac patients at St. Luke's Hospital in Missouri.[8] Dr Harris and his research team examined the health outcomes of nearly one thousand heart patients at St. Luke's Hospital. Half of the participants received daily prayer for four weeks from five Christian volunteers who believed in God and in the healing power of prayer. Harris concluded that those in the prayer group fared 11 percent better than the no-prayer group in terms of incidences of chest pains, pneumonia, infection, and death.

If you dislike the idea of praying or asking God for help, think of it as asking 'a power higher than you' to assist. Believe it or not, this could work. In fact, researchers at the University of Cologne have proven that having a superstition or just having something to believe in—even a lucky charm—can improve your self-efficacy and ability to perform in a certain task.[9] Many of my patients coming to therapy for drug addiction don't like the idea of praying or going to Alcoholics Anonymous because of the religious connotations. More often than not, the same patients who complained about this ended up benefitting from the belief in a higher power.

Why does believing in a higher power work? The reason is that 'detachment' occurs; when you put your trust or faith in something, you let go of the fear that you will not get what you want. You let go of doubt. When you are detached, you allow yourself to feel, think, and go about your life as if you already have what you want. You will feel your doubt and fear transform into a deep sense of knowing. Having that certainty is having faith. To have faith does not mean you sit back and wish things could be different. It is when you have faith that you become relaxed in the knowledge that your choice has already manifested in the mental realm from which all things manifest. Once you trust that the outcome you wish for will happen, you will automatically take inspired action toward that specific outcome. Faith means you let go of the belief 'it's not possible'. If, on the other hand, you feel a sense of panic or feel a need to control the process, then you are in doubt and disbelief. This, in turn, makes you focus on failure.

What you resist persists

Thus, to maintain that confidence that it will indeed happen, you let go of resistance and detach. Detachment is not the same as quitting. Detachment just means you longer have to worry that what you wish for will or will not come true. That's how the belief in a higher power and prayer can help.

Another example of this detachment process is of a patient who came to me for therapy distressed about not being able to fall pregnant. She had come to the point at which she had given up on it. I asked her how she would feel if she did fall pregnant. She replied, of course, 'I'd be ecstatic!' So, we spoke about that need to detach and feel ecstatic whether or not she fell pregnant. I asked her what she would be doing if she did fall pregnant. She stated she would go on holiday. So, I advised her to go on holiday and focus on feeling ecstatic. She did, and then of course the pressure was off and she fell pregnant!

How this detachment process applies to your weight loss is this: if you are anxious about not achieving your weight management goal, you will be stressed. Stress elevates your cortisol (stress hormones) which will prevent weight loss. Once you let go, it will happen easily because the pressure is off.

'What the mind can conceive and believe, it can achieve.' (Napoleon Hill)

To improve your self-efficacy, do at least one the following:

The Eight 'I Can Do This' Exercises

'I can do this' exercise 1: Remind yourself of your previous successes

Think back to a time you were able to achieve any of the goals you are currently wanting to achieve. For example, if you want to avoid going for second helpings after dinner, think back to a time that you managed to do that. Identify how you did this.

'I can do this' exercise 2: Just try, then persist

Identify something you would like to achieve in terms of your weight management goal. Today: just attempt it. Whether or not you succeed is irrelevant. Just try it. If you do not succeed, just try again tomorrow. If you do succeed, do it again ... and again.

'I've been on a diet for 2 weeks and all I've lost is 2 weeks.' (Totie Fields)

'I can do this' exercise 3: Replace 'I can't' with 'I can'

Reprogram your mind with powerful self-talk. You can do this by replacing the words 'I can't' with a phrase that is more empowering. Instead of saying, 'I can't,' say, 'I don't (yet).' For example, instead of, 'I can't stop eating the wrong foods/I can't eat chocolate/exercise/lose weight,' say, 'I don't eat chocolate.' For things you need to do, but do not yet believe you can do, practice saying, 'I am in the process of learning how to how to eat in moderation/waking up at 6am to exercise.'

'I can do this' exercise 4: Transfer your skills

Step 1: Identify a goal you have had in the past. A financial, career, or educational goal, other personal goal, relationship goal, etc. How did you go about succeeding in it? Apply these same principles to your weight loss goal.

Step 2: Identify how you can apply these strategies to your weight loss goal.

'I can do this' exercise 5: Why I can

Look at a photo of yourself at your current weight and/or weigh yourself. Then follow these steps:

Step 1: Set a timer for 4 minutes. In those 4 minutes write down all the reasons you would like to be slim/normalise your eating.

Step 2: Set a timer for 4 minutes. Write down all the reasons you CAN be slim/normalise your eating.

'I can do this' exercise 6: Get inspiration from the ones who have overcome adversity

Think of a person you know (a colleague, neighbour, friend, relative, TV actress, or TV personality, etc.) who has succeeded with the goal you would like to achieve. For example, a friend who lost 10kg by going to the gym every day. Identify how he or she was able to do this. You may also feel inspired by the success stories and the support you can get from other members of Overeaters Anonymous meetings. You can also look at YouTube for weight loss success stories or other online success stories although be aware that not all of them are genuine (some may be people advertising a specific weight loss product). The National Weight Control Registry may also inspire. But apart from weight loss per se, you may also find yourself getting inspired by reading any of the following books and/or watch suggested TV shows, even if they are not specifically related to weight management:

Book suggestions:

True Spirit by Jessica Watson

Never Stop Believing by Sally Obermeder

Disarm Your Limits by Jessica Cox

Limitless by Nick Vujicic

Rise by Ingrid Poulson

Everything to Live For by Turia Pitt

The Magic of Believing by Claude Bristol

The Success Principles by Jack Canfield

www.jackcanfield.com

The Silva Method www.silvamethod.com.au

TV show suggestions:

'Dynamo: Magician Impossible', anything by Derren Brown, 'Extreme Makeover Weight Loss Edition' by Chris Powell

‘I can do this’ exercise 7: Ask for help

If God is a part of your life, pray for help with your eating/weight issue, otherwise, request help from a higher power.

‘I can do this’ exercise 8: Use hypnosis to improve your self-efficacy

Of course, you may also know that just like sports psychologists who use hypnosis to improve athletes’ sports performance to increase their self-efficacy, you too can use the power of hypnosis to improve your self-efficacy to achieve your ideal body and more harmonious eating behaviours. You will find more details in the hypnosis chapter, but bear in mind the above strategies are also very powerful.

Chapter 3: **Feeding Your Self-Esteem, Not Your Stomach**

'Confidence is contagious. So is lack of confidence.'
(Vince Lombardi)

Gain Self-Esteem to Lose Your Unwanted Body Hatred/Fat and Urge to Binge/Overeat

When your self-esteem is high, it means you generally evaluate yourself positively. When your self-esteem is low, you are likely to judge yourself negatively and may be self-conscious, shy or very sensitive to criticism. If you chronically put yourself down with thoughts such as 'I'm not good enough', or 'I'm so stupid', your confidence in yourself and your ability to succeed will be compromised. This chapter will help you demolish those and build up your self-esteem. Why is self-esteem so important in getting control of your eating and weight? Research has proven that:

- Poor self-esteem is associated with emotional eating[1]
- Fad dieting, and its almost inevitable failure and link with bingeing/overeating, breaks down self-esteem[2]

- The more critical you are about yourself, the worse your eating disorder[3]
- The more diets you have been on, the worse your self-esteem[3]

It should not be surprising to you to learn that failing again and again can damage self-esteem. But if you are like most people, you will have been on diet after diet, trying one slimming program after another, attributing the 'failure' (not being able to adhere to a slimming diet), on your own inadequacies rather than on external factors beyond your control. You delve into guilt and shame and lose even more confidence. Guilt, shame, and loss of confidence then leads to lack of self-care. Some people who come to my office with reports of having struggled with their weight, don't realise how badly they treat themselves. I hear a fairly similar story of self-neglect to which you may be able to relate:

> 'I don't have time to prepare proper meals. Sometimes I don't get time to eat so I eat on the run. I don't have time to cook. We just have a microwave meal or a take-away because I couldn't be bothered to cut up vegetables. I will eat anything I can get that's quick: a pie, a packet of chips, burgers and chips, a family-sized chocolate block. I just don't have the time: I get up, drive an hour to work, work for 10 hours, then drive home for an hour, and then go to bed. Who has time to cook meals or prepare a salad? I don't have time to exercise because I work all day, come home, help the kids with homework, cook dinner, rush the meal, clean up, get barely enough sleep, and do it all again the next day.'

If you can relate to the above example, focusing on work, housework, and everything and everyone except yourself, neglecting your diet and personal needs, there's probably a part of you that knows that following this protocol is not working for you weight, your body image, nor your self-esteem. But how do you change that? How do you not do this? How do you take time out so that you can look after yourself? There's probably a part of you that knows you need to nurture yourself and stop criticising yourself, but another part that keeps on doing the same thing and expecting different results.

If those two parts of you had a chat to each other, would one of them say, 'That's just crazy! I know that my weight/eating problem is because I neglect and abuse myself by not eating right and not exercising. I'm now also being bullied by an employer, abused by a partner, teased by classmates or siblings, or degraded by parents!' The good news is that *Weight Off Your Mind* will help you find a better balance. Imagine a life in which you nurture yourself with a healthy diet and exercise and in turn be a good role model to your children or peers or colleagues ... the other good news is that your family, your colleagues, your peers, and everyone around you will benefit too.

> Events—whether self-induced or triggered by others—that instil or perpetuate the beliefs: 'I'm insignificant, I'm a failure, I cannot succeed, I'm stupid, I'm not good enough/inadequate, I'm not worthy' will negatively affect your self-esteem and are likely to perpetuate your weight management problems.

How so? I had a patient who was a mother of a five-year-old boy. She was a dedicated mother. She called off a doctor's appointment because she felt guilty about making him miss his play date with his friend if she did go to her Dr's appointment. When we discussed this, she identified that she had put off the doctor's appointment already for several months. She complained of constant fatigue and knew she needed to get to the bottom of this, but she couldn't put herself first. She was never her own priority. When she finally made alternative arrangements for her son, and put herself first by attending the doctor's appointment, it was a very simple solution. She found out she was iron-deficient, started taking iron tablets, then had the energy to exercise and consequently had decreased hunger and decreased weight almost instantly! Of course, as a loving mother, she was also pleased to report she had more energy to play with him! She recognised that by taking care of herself first she could be an even better mother. But this example applies even if you're not a mother. It applies to you if you have ever neglected yourself in order to take care of other people or things *at your expense* and consequently moved you further away from your slimming goal.

Have you ever neglected yourself because you felt you had to put others or work first?

If you thought of your body as your own child, what kind of love, care, attention, and nurturing would you give it? If you have ever listened to the emergency instruction on a plane, you would have heard the hostess saying, 'In case of emergency, oxygen masks will drop down. Please fit the masks on *yourself* before fitting them onto your children.'

Whenever I've heard this announcement, I've always been confused. But then it was clear: how can you help your children, if you yourself cannot breathe?

What do you plan to do differently now that you know you need to make space for self-care?

Love Your Body—It Will Love You Back

The above section alerted you to the idea that you need to take care of yourself first before taking care of your loved ones and work. However, another way that you may have been damaging your self-esteem is by neglecting to value yourself by focusing on criticising your appearance. If you tend to look at your body (or parts of it) and react with, 'Ugh! Disgusting,' or similar, you may also notice that you also tend to focus a great deal on what other people look like. If you constantly think of yourself as fat (or similar), you may also be in the habit of comparing yourself to other people. This comparison, 'I should not look like this. I should be more like … ' is one of the most damaging thing you can do to your self-esteem and therefore is something that sabotages your slimming journey rather than enhances it. In fact, research has provided evidence that people with Binge Eating Disorders overvalue the importance of shape and weight.[4]

> Research has proven that the more important you believe shape/weight is, the worse your eating behaviour is.[4]

Imagine for a moment that you focused on other wonderful qualities about yourself rather than on your body/appearance/shape … imagine paying attention to other things in your life that are important … imagine that instead of blaming and criticising yourself, you continually love yourself unconditionally like you love your family, pets or friends? Countless studies have identified that in order to end problematic eating, self-compassion needs to replace self-blame. In fact, Canadian researchers found that women who have low self-compassion were more likely to have eating disorders and that improving self-compassion is an important part in recovery.[5] Therefore, exercises to decrease shame and self-critical thoughts are likely to lift you out of that negativity.[6] It's time right now to let go of negativity and embrace love and greater self-esteem. Love yourself enough to do at least one of:

The Ten Pathways to Loving Your Body Into Slimness

Love your body slim pathway #1: Change negative self-talk

Become aware of negative self-talk, then stop it. Identify today how often you put yourself down. For example, when you make a mistake, do you say, 'I'm such an idiot?' If so, be aware of it and make a change so that you talk to yourself as you would talk to your best friend. For example, say, 'So, I've made a mistake, that's okay. I have learned from this. I'm still okay. I am still good enough. I am still worthy.'

Love your body slim pathway #2: Change negative 'body' talk

Catch yourself every time you are critical about your body. Then talk to your body (or body part that you particularly dislike) as though it is your best friend, e.g. 'I love you despite your faults; I accept you as you are.' Imagine that you separated your self-worth from your weight/shape. How would you feel? What other qualities do you have?

> Evaluating yourself as 'bad' for eating a certain food is the best way to stay fat and perpetuate problem eating.

Stop body checking and comparing yourself with others. Remember that models and actresses in magazines have their photos retouched and are therefore NOT accurate images of a 'perfect' body. If this is a major problem for you, spend some time with the exercises in the later chapter 'Body Image'.

Love your body slim pathway #4: Avoid negative people

Imagine your life if you spring cleaned your life of people who frequently upset you, sabotage your success, criticise you, or use you. The first step is to identify any and all abusers whether it's the boss, your work colleagues, your relatives/in-laws, or your so-called 'friends' by identifying what it is that they are doing that sabotage your success: for example, you have told someone you are on a weight loss mission and are currently avoiding chocolate, but this person gives you chocolates for your birthday; or someone who makes you run errands all the time, making you miss your exercise session. I understand that it may not be possible to remove yourself from all of these sabotagers or abusers. If you cannot avoid them, make a plan to assert yourself with your abusers/sabotagers. If you find yourself in a position of being used a great deal by others, decide today whether this is helpful or not. If it's working against you and your slimming goal, pledge as of today to respond differently. Whenever somebody asks you to do something, identify if you are doing it for approval or whether you are doing it for genuine reasons. Pledge to do something for someone only if it's mutually beneficial rather than simply to get approval (especially if you do not like the person). Letting go of or finding a better way to cope with people who chronically (or even occasionally) abuse you can be a difficult process. If you are struggling with this, discuss it with your therapist.

Love your body slim pathway #5: Assert yourself

When you are a door-mat, people will walk all over you. If you assert yourself—whether it's food related or not—you will gain respect and your body will thank you for it too. If you are struggling to assert yourself, discuss it in therapy with your psychologist. Know your bill of rights. Never, ever eat (more) simply to please someone or avoid displeasing someone. Refusing an offer of (more) food is not rude. It's your right. Think of it as someone offering chocolate to a diabetic. You can just say no.

Love your body slim pathway #6: Accept positive feedback

Whenever you get a compliment, accept it. Start by just responding with, 'Thank you!'

Love your body slim pathway #7: Ask others for help

Do you value yourself enough to ask others to help you? Example: ask your partner or your teenagers to do the cooking, laundry, or other household tasks.

Love your body slim pathway #8: Remind yourself how wonderful you truly have been and are

Imagine if you walked into a room that was full of people who reminded you of everything you've ever felt ashamed about, guilty about, depressed about ... how would you feel? My guess is that you would feel ashamed, guilty, and depressed! But this is what you may be doing at the moment with your own thoughts. Thus, remove that negative picture. Instead imagine walking into a room that is full of people who reminded you of everything you've ever done that made you feel proud, happy, and fulfilled. Whereas this may not be possible in real life, one way you can anchor positivity in your life is to keep reminders around your home and work environment of how wonderful you are: this could be through photographs of friends or family members you love, thank you cards you have received, certificates—anything that puts you in a positive mindset.

Love your body slim pathway #9: Participate in a self-esteem workshop (live or through manuals)

If you are struggling to love your body and build up your self-esteem, inquire about an assertiveness or self-esteem workshop, or check out these resources:

Helpful resources:

www.cci.health.wa.gov.au ('Assert Yourself and Improving Your Self-Esteem')

The Science of Self-Confidence by Brian Tracy

Say No Without Feeling Guilty by Patti Breitman and Connie Hatch

The Compassionate Mind Approach to Beating Overeating by Dr Ken Goss

Love your body slim pathway #10: Use hypnosis and other mind-power methods

You will find that EMDR, hypnosis, and other mind power methods in this book are able to assist you in improving your self-esteem. For example, EMDR is a method that alleviates the damage done by a critical parent who instilled guilt or shame in you.

Chapter 4: **Slimming by Social Osmosis**

'You are the average of the 5 people you spend the most time with.'
(Jim Rohn)

As you're reading this book and wondering how this all works, you will notice that you keep getting ideas about how to make losing weight and keeping it off a much easier process. A study published in the *American Journal of Clinical Nutrition* found one of the differences between relapsers and maintainers was that 70 percent of maintainers used available social support.[1] The same was found by two other major investigations into what makes people lose weight and maintain weight loss.[2] No other weight management book will reveal this magic trick. This chapter provides you with the secret ingredient that will facilitate weight management for you:

Slimming by Osmosis Tip 1: Many Helping Hands Make Light Body

In a systematic review of 30 studies which investigated diet and exercise interventions, the researchers concluded that one of the things that enhances interventions is social support.[3] The power of social support has also been evident in treatment of other disorders including cancer—studies have shown that survival rates are much higher if social support is strong.[4] Dr James Fowler of the University of California (San Diego), who researched the influence of our social network on weight, discovered that if you go on a diet with a friend (of the same gender), you have a greater chance of success than if you do it alone.[5]

Social support can also be in the form of telling other people about your weight loss goal—research has supported the hypothesis that the more people you tell about your goal, the more likely it is that you will achieve it.[6] Evidence of the benefits of social support to slim down was also found in a study of 633 people who had better outcomes when social support was provided to navigate social undermining of healthy eating and physical activity.[7]

Research at the University of Waterloo in Canada discovered that when people are supported by others with positive messages about their weight tend to lose weight, whereas those who receive critical feedback about their weight tend to gain weight.[8]

Another study published in *Obesity* even found that peer support worked as effectively as professional support when it comes to weight loss.[9] Peer support is, however, most effective when the people providing support are themselves successful in losing weight.[10] That is the reason Overeaters Anonymous can be so helpful. I had a colleague who told me she had lost 12kg in 3 months with the support of an online

30-day no sugar challenge. For example, if you prefer to receive internet support, you can do that. However, bear in mind that most research has found face-to-face, especially group support, is better than online support.[11]

The idea of being supported by an expert, i.e. 'learning on the job', should be a familiar one. As mentioned in the self-efficacy chapter, a mentor is so crucial in your weight management goal, not only to boost your self-efficacy but also to provide you with the understanding, 'I know what you're going through and I can help you.' There's only so much you can do by yourself and learn from a book—the rest you absorb from those who do it naturally. Mentors are crucial to remind you of the stuff books don't tell you, guide you when there's an exception, motivate you to do something you've never done before, provide you with confidence of being able to achieve your goal, to correct you when you've made a mistake, to nurture you along the way, and to praise you when you've done something well.

You may also be familiar with the Alcoholics Anonymous (A.A.) model of 'learn from the ones who've done it'. In my clinical practice, I've had many patients who have benefitted a great deal from the whole group as well as their sponsors (people with long term sobriety). In psychological treatments, several studies have found that group treatments may produce larger weight losses than individual programs.[12] Support groups including Overeaters Anonymous (O.A.) may be helpful specifically because they are run by people who are also in recovery from overeating. As in Alcoholics Anonymous, senior members in Overeaters Anonymous provide valuable support to others also struggling with overeating.

The founder of Overeaters Anonymous Rozanne made a wonderful promise to her meeting attendees: 'I put my hand in yours and together we can do what we could never do alone.' If you are like most of my patients who dislike the idea of needing somebody and asking for help, think again. Think about the last time you achieved something great. Did you achieve it alone or with somebody's help? If you have been stuck for years, struggling by yourself with your weight/eating war, give yourself the gift of asking at least one person for help. Ditch the idea of not wanting to bother or burden anybody else. The idea of being able to conquer something big like your weight problem alone is lofty. Have you achieved your weight goal without somebody's help before? Do you know anybody who has? Your weight/eating goal is unlikely to happen unless you ask for help. If it does happen without anyone's help, please let me know. In all my fourteen years of clinical practice, I've not seen anybody overcome a problem without the help of someone: family members, friends, sponsors, a therapist, others in a support group, or neighbours. Remember: together you can make magic happen.

'Alone we can do so little; together we can do so much.' (*Deaf-blind political activist and author Helen Keller*)

Researchers investigated the impact of social support on weight loss and maintenance.[13] They recruited participants either alone or as a group with three friends and randomly assigned them to one of two groups who received either standard behavioural treatment or standard behavioural treatment plus social support. They found that participants recruited with friends and those who were in the standard behavioural treatment plus social support group, demonstrated improved weight loss and weight maintenance: 66 percent maintained their weight loss in full. Those with social support were also more likely to complete the ten-month program—retention rate was 95 percent!

Another study of 198 overweight and obese adolescents, examined the impact of perceived social support in weight management.[14] The results indicated that those who perceived their friends as supportive not only reported confidence in their ability to succeed, but also achieved greater weight losses.

Having worked in the addiction field for over 15 years, I have been so drawn to what Johann Hari said about addiction. Although he was talking about drug addiction specifically, I believe it applies to food addiction too. Hari stated: 'The opposite of addiction is not sobriety. The opposite of addiction is connection.' I highly recommend reading his very inspirational insight—either by reading an article in the Huffington Post or reading his book *Chasing The Scream*.

My personal experience of writing *Weight Off Your Mind* could not have been achieved without the motivation I received from my success coaches Jodie and Peter Conna, all 96 participants and staff at the Life Design, my patients who provided me with the opportunity to help them, and my business mentor Angela Raspass. My own weight loss could not have been achieved without the support of my therapist, my professors, my friends, and books I had read.

Ask for support

- ✓ Ask at least one friend and/or colleague to join you on your mission to normalise your eating and achieve your weight management goal
- ✓ Tell as many people as possible about your weight loss goal
- ✓ Find a mentor (someone who has achieved a weight loss goal) and spend as much time with him or her as possible
- ✓ Join a Facebook or online thirty-day support group or start your own. If you're not a social media fan, google 'weight loss challenge' or similar to access one of many inspiring stories and valuable support online
- ✓ Join Overeaters Anonymous in group or online: www.Avision4you.org

Slimming by Osmosis Tip 2: Eat With the Right People

Researchers have proven that your commitment to a health/weight loss goal can be influenced by the people with whom you eat.[15] A research team at the Southern Illinois University found that eating a meal in the presence of an overweight person, particularly one who serves him or herself unhealthy food, increases the likelihood of you eating unhealthy food. In addition, it also makes a difference what sort of partner you choose: apparently, your chance of becoming obese increases 37 percent if your partner is obese.[16] Conversely, the opposite is also true: if you eat with a slim person, you are more likely to eat less. Another study has found that if a woman dines with a man she will eat about 100 calories less than when she dines with a female.[17]

Eat with slim people

✓ To ease your slimming journey, as much as possible, eat with people who are slim, or are on the weight loss journey with you

Slimming by Osmosis Tip 3: Socialise With Slim People

You may be familiar with the saying: 'you are what you eat'. I believe there is a far more fitting one: 'you are who you spend most time with'. Research by Dr James Fowler has found that you are 40 percent more likely to be obese if your friends are obese, and even if your friend's friend is obese, even if you live very far away from each other.[18] This does not mean 'dump your fat friends.' Rather, because of the influence you would have losing weight, you will not only affect a friend who wants to lose weight, but also a friend's friend. I have personally experienced two of my friends losing weight shortly after I achieved my weight loss goal—and I, of course, lost weight, following my friend's weight loss.

'If you want to go fast, go alone; if you want to go far, go together.' (African proverb)

Self-made millionaire and author Jim Rohn says, 'you are the average of the five people you spend the most time with.' If you were to list the five people with whom you spend the most time, would you say you have friends fatter than you and friends slimmer than you? One way to improve your chances of success to achieve your ideal body—as simple as it seems—is to add another one, two, or three or more slim people into your life. In other words, it's almost like slimming down by virtue of spending time with them.

Twelve step programs like Narcotics Anonymous have a saying: 'if you're going to the barber shop, you're gonna get a haircut'. This means if you are going to be around other drug users or hang out in drug venues (nightclubs, crack houses), you will eventually use drugs. I believe the same is true for weight related issues. If you are around people who eat junk all the time, you're more likely to do the same, whereas if you socialise with slim people who may have a more active lifestyle and eat healthier, it is likely to influence you.

If you're around people at the moment who have weight problems, offer to take them on the weight loss journey with you. If they don't want to at the moment, don't push them. You can be there for them when they're ready. But if you come up against negativity, consider 'detoxing' your life of people who don't support you. Think of it as a spring clean of people who bring you down. Instead, seek out people who support you and treat you with kindness and love. Bear in mind that a powerful attachment with another person can actually change your nervous system.[19] You cannot afford to expose yourself to toxic relationships any more than you should take drugs and not expect the entire brain to be profoundly impacted.

Spend time with slim people

Spend time in places where you can meet slim people, e.g. go to a gym and speak to people there or join bushwalking groups and walk with the slim ones, strike up a conversation, then a friendship. Ensure that the people you spend time with treat you with kindness, love, and respect.

Exercise for enthusiasts:

Break through the politically correctness of not mentioning the 'elephant in the room.' Most people who are overweight or obese find the term 'fat' offensive. Saying to someone, 'You're fat,' is inappropriate only because it is perceived as a dirty word. However, saying, 'You're diabetic,' is as factual yet not offensive. Most obese and overweight people know that they are 'fat' but denial of it keeps them overeating or bingeing. It prevents them from taking—in some cases—necessary steps to save their lives or at least improve their health and energy. If someone (even your own GP) had pointed out to you that your weight is problematic to your health, would you have taken steps or even thought about making changes?

If you have a 'fat' friend, colleague, neighbour, or relative, offer them support to lose the weight. Perhaps approach it with, for example, 'Let's do it together.' If you don't offer others support, who will give them the wake up call? The emergency room doctor? I'm not suggesting you walk up to someone and say, 'Gee, you're fat. You need to lose weight.' Rather, I'm suggesting to approach the matter gently and diplomatically with someone who is likely to be open to receiving help. For example, you may talk about your own problem with weight and say, 'How do you feel about your weight?' If the response is something you can work with, go further by saying, 'I'm in the process of losing weight. Would you be interested in doing it together?'

Chapter 5: **Stress Management for Slimming**

'People often say that motivation doesn't last. Well, neither does bathing—that's why we recommend it daily.'
(Motivational speaker Zig Ziglar)

Throughout my years as a hypnotherapist, I've had hundreds of people phone me up to request a hypnosis session to lose weight. I always do a thorough assessment and more often than not, the person sitting in front of me is someone who has recently gone through multiple stressors. When I say to them that I recommend they address these stressors first, some of them will insist, 'No, thanks, I just want the hypnosis so I can lose weight.' What these people are really saying is, 'Please just fix me quickly. I'm going through enough and I just want the weight to be gone so I have one thing less to worry about.'

My response to this is usually, 'Okay, I will do the hypnosis because you have requested it. I will give you the very best hypnosis session I know. However, just know that the chances of you accelerating your response to this session is much lower than if you deal with the stressors first.' To my surprise, in some cases, the hypnosis session without dealing with the stressors has actually worked! However, in most cases, the person comes back the following session, complaining about it working at first but not lasting or working only at 50 percent capacity.

Hypnosis is a magic wand but it doesn't make the stressors in your life disappear. Fortunately, finding a way to cope with the stressor is the magic wand needed to accelerate the results of the hypnosis. An example of how applying simple stress management skills can make you lose weight is that of a patient who was struggling and 'stressed' because her in-laws were living with her and, amongst other things, annoyed her because they did not help her with the housework. We spent a whole session working out how to cope with this stressor without even doing hypnosis. She came to me three weeks later, requesting another hypnosis session even though she had already lost 2kg just by using communication skills (we had discussed) with them.

Manage Stress, Manage Abdominal Fat

It should be no surprise to you that whereas some people don't eat more when they are stressed, most overweight and obese people tend to eat more when they are stressed. In fact, this was proven in a study that found that 'high cortisol reactors' consumed more calories and more sweet food when stressed, especially if their mood was depressed.[1] Research has also confirmed:

- We tend to eat more sugar and fat, i.e. 'comfort foods', when stressed to reduce anxiety[2]
- A major study of 12,110 people found that those who had high stress levels had a high fat diet[3]
- We tend to have increased appetite during times of stress due to the increase in the stress hormone cortisol[4]

- Work stress increases weight in already overweight men[5]

Psychological causes of stress eating

Kaplan and Kaplan's psychosomatic theory of obesity in 1957 postulated that because eating can reduce anxiety, people learn to eat when anxious, resulting in compulsive eating.[6]

Stress Defined: 'Stressed' is Desserts Spelled Backwards!

Life does not always work out as you want it to. You feel stressed and eat desserts, right? What is stress anyway? Stress is different things to different people. You may worry about the health of family members or pets; have car problems on a day you really need the car; have arguments with a partner or your ex-partner, relative, neighbours, a friend, colleagues, or your boss; you may be upset about the traffic, the weather, house renovations, financial worries, all your responsibilities or being lonely. You may have work-related problems including feeling unfulfilled, bullied, underpaid, undervalued or under time pressure. You may find yourself stressed due to an illness or pain or worry about other aspects of your appearance, such as ageing. Stress can also be linked to a positive thing including planning a wedding or journey.

Any of the above mentioned stressors may affect you at different levels than another person and also compared to other times in your life you may have experienced a similar stressor. For example, you may find that what stressed you ten years ago may not stress you currently. Or you may find yourself perplexed about why you are stressed about something that other people don't find stressful. It also seems that if you are a woman, you're more likely to stress-eat compared to a man.[7]

Thus, it is not the event itself that is stressful, it is your perception of that particular event. For example, during the 2013 bushfires in the Blue Mountains, some people directly affected by the bushfires brushed it off with a simple, 'material things can be replaced', whereas others, who weren't even directly affected, had serious psychological and even physical symptoms of stress. We know for example that peptic ulcers are caused by stress,[8] as is IBS [9]and even heart disease.[10]

Stress can vary from day to day and from week to week too. What effect is it having on your body? Is it causing you headaches or other pain? Is it making you eat on the run? Is it driving you to comfort eat? Is it causing your sleep to be disrupted? Is it making you short-tempered? Is it affecting your relationship? Stress affects people in different ways. Some people—like you—may binge eat to comfort and sedate. Quite incredibly, some people lose their appetite when they're stressed! Other people cope by avoiding or escaping a situation whereas others engage in problem solving. Some people ruminate, increasing their use of drugs, cigarettes, or alcohol, whereas others engage in healthy coping skills. For some people, it may be second nature to engage in destructive coping skills whereas others will engage in healthy coping skills to deal with stress. You may find that sometimes you engage in healthy coping skills, like talking to a friend about a problem, whereas at other times you binge eat or engage in other destructive coping skills.

When you are unable to balance out your stress with coping skills, your body will then feel the effect of stress. According to brain studies, stress can actually shrink parts of the brain.[11] The brain is certainly not something we want to shrink. If you want your fat rather than your brain to shrink, here are further reasons to manage your stress.

> The more stressed you feel, the less weight you lose[12]

5 Reasons Managing Your Stress Will Help You Manage Your Weight

1. Manage stress, manage abdominal fat

A study published in the journal *Psychoneuroendocrinology* reported that stress has been linked to increased abdominal fat due to repeated activation of the stress hormone cortisol. Stress eating may also increase visceral fat even without weight gain. Visceral fat is body fat that is stored within the abdominal cavity, around the liver, pancreas, and intestines,[13] and therefore is the fat that is also linked to illnesses. Thus, if you manage your stress, you're also preventing major illnesses related to fat accumulation.

2. Manage stress, manage hormone levels

If your hormones are not balanced, you are likely to experience increased hunger, increased desire to eat sweets, and generally increased food intake.[14]

3. Manage stress, manage nutritional balance

Research has shown that stress draws out vital vitamins and nutrients.[15] This, in turn, could make you feel tired. When tired, you may eat sugary foods to lift your energy. Or you may eat more food to get enough nutrients.

4. Manage stress, manage attraction to fatty, salty and sugary foods

According to an article in *Appetite*, stressed-out eaters were more likely to consume fatty, salty, and sugary foods.[16] Thus, it makes sense to de-stress to de-grease!

5. Manage stress, manage binge eating

According to research, binge eaters tend to have a deficit in stress management skills. The good news, however, is that you can learn to manage your stress[17] which, in turn, decreases your tendency to binge eat.

Melt Away Your Stress With Any of the 5 Power Methods

A variety of different stress management methods are available. Yoga and meditation are just two of many options. A few interesting methods have recently emerged: research at the University College London noted that people who drank black tea four times a day for six weeks had lower levels of cortisol after a stressful task than those who drank a caffeinated fruit beverage.[18] A seemingly simple thing like drinking tea, you ask? Well, a study at Swinburne University of Technology found even chewing gum while anxious reduced stress by 17 percent.[19] However, tea drinking and gum chewing are not very well supported stress management methods. Although I would not discourage tea drinking or gum chewing necessarily, methods with more scientific support outlined below may be more helpful. I have a friend who attributes her mental health to Ayurvedic and Chinese herbs including Korean ginseng, rhodiola, ashwagandha (withania), licorice, cordyceps mushrooms, and magnolia. Herbs however—although popular in the alternative medicine field—have not had a great deal of scientific support. My other friend prefers mindfulness methods, which are of course backed up with a great deal of scientific evidence. Do whatever works for you.

The following is a list of methods that can help to reduce stress and therefore help you achieve your weight management goal. You will see in other chapters the magic stress reduction power of getting enough sleep and exercising. The stress management methods that work for me include getting adequate sleep, managing my time, having pets, a weekly massage, listening to music, lots of laughter, exercising, and meditating. Find the ones that work for you. You may find that a combination of methods achieves the best results. Stress management is something you should practice daily. If you think you can skip your stress management exercise (whether that's meditation, yoga, talking to friends, etc.), because you don't think it will work/affect you if you don't do it, remember: stress will always have a negative consequence to your life and your weight/eating.

Stress melting, fat melting power method #1: Balance your work/play time

Have you heard of 'all work and no play makes Jack a dull boy?' It's true that good time management leads to effortless weight management. If you find yourself continually rushing or having difficulty with energy and motivation, you're most likely in need of time management strategies. Once you master your time, you will find that you're more able to be more productive at work, be more attentive with your spouse and kids, and of course, achieve your weight loss goal.

Time management involves finding a balance between things you have to do (e.g. paying household bills, doing household chores, and working) and things you want to do. If your only pleasure is derived from eating food, your body is going to ache for something to do instead if you suddenly quit deriving it from bingeing. If you don't know what to do for fun, find something you used to do (e.g. writing), something your colleagues do (e.g. candle making), something your friend does (e.g. taking a language course), something your relative does (e.g. knitting), or something you have always wanted to do (e.g. skydiving, going to see a stand-up comedy show). Even a simple thing like reading for just six minutes, for example, can reduce stress levels by 68 percent, according to research at the University of Sussex.[20]

I had a patient who attended weight management sessions with me after she gained weight after quitting smoking three months before. She stated she had used cigarettes to 'take a break' and now had 'no excuse to go out and take a break' and found herself eating to make up for it. We discussed starting a hobby. Though reluctant to start, she decided to do art, and of course, lost interest in bingeing because she was too busy drawing things.

I would recommend time management books including *Time Management for Dummies* (Clare Evans), getting help from a professional organiser, or sticking to the main time management strategies: writing things in a calendar, minimising time wasters, delegating tasks others can do, and doing things while you're waiting (e.g. in a queue). Stress management classes can also be helpful. A holiday—even just a weekend away—can also do wonders. I've also found that patients report that my advice to limit TV or Facebook time to 2 hours maximum per day is helpful.

Stress melting, fat melting power method #2: Meditate

Meditation was one of the major elements that changed my life for the better. I have practiced Transcendental Meditation (TM) since 1991. I must admit, there have been times when I did not practice it at all for a few weeks, even months. Yet, whenever I practice it again, I feel the benefits right away. I feel calmer, happier, find myself making lucky discoveries, need one hour less sleep, meet the right people, and achieve better results with my patients.

When I started Dr Dyer's meditation in 2008, I wanted to emulate him in terms of meditating to get something specific—a kind of wish fulfilment meditation. I thought I'd start with something simple. So, I meditated on the idea that I needed a cutting tool to cut five vinyl tiles. I didn't want to have to go to the shop to buy a cutter just to cut those five vinyl tiles so I thought, *Why not try and see what happens?* So I did and the very next day I found a cutter lying on the street just as I was walking my dog! I thought, *This is amazing!*

I had done a similar thing many years previously. I had been speaking to a lady who told me that she had been given a bouquet of flowers by a stranger on Valentine's Day. I was so jealous, I really wanted that to happen to me too. So, I meditated on this and indeed, I did get a bouquet on Valentine's from a stranger! If you think that meditation is just some airy-fairy thing that new age hippies do, think again—meditation is useful for managing bingeing too.

It is quite possible that even if you do only meditation (and nothing else in *Weight Off Your Mind*) that you will achieve your weight loss goal.

Several studies have proven that meditation can assist in alleviating the urge to binge eat.[21] Dr Sara Lazar, a leading neuroscientist and meditation researcher at the Massachussets General Hospital and Harvard Medical School, has focused her research on the neuro-biological underpinnings of meditation. She has been able to identify how meditation changes the brain using magnetic resonance imaging (MRI). If you would like to find out more about this fascinating field, you can go to www.lazar-meditation-research.info or source any of Dr Meares' books, such as *Relief Without Drugs.*

Apart from reducing stress hormones prolactin and glucocorticoids, meditation has also been found to lower thyroid-stimulating hormone (TSH) that prevents depression and increases serotonin levels, which improves your mood.[22] These effects are likely to help you alleviate binge eating as the underlying reasons for overeating and bingeing are uprooted. I have had several of my patients report not bingeing on the days they meditate! It can be quite profound. However, if you don't get such immediate results, do not give up. Meditation appears to have a cumulative effect—you will derive long term benefits from practicing it regularly.

If you have never meditated and wonder what it is like, before you think that meditation is not for you because you are unable to sit still, concentrate, ponder, and be quiet, you should know that's actually not what meditation is. Meditation causes you to be quiet. It doesn't require you to concentrate and certainly shouldn't involve stressing about 'not getting it right'. Just try it, don't fret; it will get easier and you will find yourself craving it. Find out which type of meditation appeals to you most. I personally like Dr Wayne Dyers' meditation, as well as Transcendental Meditation (TM). However, you can also try Mindfulness-Based Stress Reduction (MBSR) Meditation, Vipassana Meditation, Taoist or Buddhist Meditation. You can access meditation by going to meditation classes, getting a meditation CD, or finding information on the internet.

Some helpful resources

Book: *In Stillness Conquer Fear,* McKinnon

CD: 'Experiencing Stillness Meditation', available on iTunes.

Websites: www.drwaynedyer.com

www.stillnessmeditation.com.au

www.meditation.org.au

www.manifestinatisse.com

www.diamonddays.com

www.spencermethod.com/meditate

www.zenworlds.com

www.meditationwithmish.com

www.josiethomson.com 'Simple Meditation for Busy People'

If you've tried meditation and find it doesn't appeal, try a different type of meditation. Don't give up on such a wonderful method. However, you can also try an alternative—a muscle relaxation exercise: www.cci.health.wa.gov.au/docs/ACF3C8D.pdf.

Or you can listen to your favourite music—research has shown that listening to your favourite music is helpful in reducing stress.[23] Try iTunes or your CD shop for music of all types.

Stress melting, fat melting power method #3: Laugh away your fat

Who says you can't have fun while losing weight? It shouldn't be surprising to you that research has shown that laughing about something is a very effective stress reduction method.[24] Several studies—like one published in the *American Journal of Medical Science*—have confirmed that laughter actually decreases cortisol, epinephrine, growth hormone, and a major dopamine catabolite which reduce stress.[25] In fact, Norman Cousins, author of *Anatomy of an Illness*, describes how he used laughter therapy (by watching old Marx Brothers movies and Candid Camera) to cure himself of an illness.[26] He said, 'laughter has an astounding rejuvenating effect on mind and body and serves as a bulletproof vest that protects you against the ravages of negative thinking.'

The website www.laughteryoga.org reports that, 'one minute of mirthful laugher is the equivalent to a 10 minute cardiac workout on a rowing machine.' Laughter Yoga drastically reduces belly fat, which is difficult to shed even with the most intense exercise regime. Just a few laughs have the capacity to exercise the mind-body. An hour of laughter can shed as many as 500 calories! There is some support in preliminary research on the positive effects of Laughter Yoga including that it not only reduces cortisol (stress hormone) but also improves assertiveness, optimism, self-regulation, optimism, acceptance, and self-awareness.[27]

Some helpful suggestions:
Check out Carl Barron at www.carlbarron.com or get his DVDs 'One Ended Stick' (Auslan version available), 'All the Stuff I've Done Before', 'Walking Down the Street', and 'Whatever Comes Next'. You can also go to live comedy shows to check out comedians, such as Paul Foote, John Bishop, Stephen K Amos, Cal Wilson, and Julia Morris.

Stress melting, fat melting power method #4: Stretch away the weight with yoga

Yoga is a practice that is more than 2500 years old. Yoga incorporates gentle exercise (stretching and structured poses called asanas), meditation and breathing practices called pranayama. The health benefits of regular yoga practice include alleviation of high blood pressure, improved posture and circulation, and of course, stress reduction.[28]

Several studies have shown that adding yoga workouts provides an added benefit for those seeking treatment for binge eating. Sponsored by the National Cancer Institute, Kristal and colleagues at the Fred Hutchinson Cancer Research Center in Seattle led a trial involving 15,500 adults. They found that practicing one 30-minute yoga session per week for at least 4 years helped people lose 5 pounds compared to those who didn't practice yoga—they gained 14 pounds. Although a typical yoga class may burn only half as many calories as walking, it can facilitate weight loss due to its effect of mind-body awareness—the ability to observe what is happening internally in a non-reactive fashion.[29]

If you have tried a particular type of yoga class before and didn't like it, rest assured they are many types from which to choose: Hatha, Anusari, Restorative, Prenatal, Vinyasa, Ashtanga, Kundalini, Inyengar, Bikram, Acroyoga, even anti-gravity, yoga from the sky, stand-up paddleboard yoga, and hip-hop yoga. Bikram Yoga involves twenty-six asanas (postures) and two breathing exercises performed over 90 minutes in a room heated to 38°C. The newer version of this is Hom Yoga performed in far infrared light, which is said to regenerate cells, heal the skin, and boost blood circulation, flexibility, and suppleness, facilitate toxin removal, and burn up to 4,200 kilojoules.

Some helpful resources

Websites: www.homyoga.com.au, www.charlotte-dodson.tv, www.EkhartYoga.com

Apps: 'Pocket Yoga' (on iTunes).

Books: *Emotional yoga: How the body can heal the mind* (Bennett); *Bringing yoga to life* (Farhi); *Yoga from the inside out: Making peace with your body* (Sell)

Stress melting, fat melting power method #5: Love, hugs, and kisses

The University of Miami Medical School's Touch Research Institute has proven in multiple studies that touch—whether through a hug or a massage—is an effective strategy to reduce stress. When I was working as a student researcher at this Institute in 1994, we were researching the effectiveness of massage on babies born prematurely due to their mothers being addicted to crack. The results were remarkable. The babies showed vast improvements in their ability to thrive.

If you've ever come through a difficult time with the help of your friends and family, you will know how comforting a loved one's hugs and kisses can be. Studies have shown the remarkable effect of human touch. At least one study has shown that frequent hugs from a partner reduces blood pressure and heart rate in people.[30] But pets also have an extraordinary effect on being able to increase serotonin and oxytocin (our feel good hormones) and decrease stress levels.[31]

If you're unable to accommodate a pet due to living in an apartment or being limited due to spending a great deal of time away from home, do your best to befriend a neighbour's or friend's pet and spend some time with that pet—whether it is for a walk or just a cuddle. For the highly enthusiastic: start a petition to prevent landlords and body corporates from banning pets in rentals.

Combination of several methods:

A study published in the *American Journal of Health Promotion* confirmed that combining different strategies of stress management is helpful.[32] More specifically, the combination of deep breathing, relaxation response, meditation, and guided imagery techniques seem to be most effective at helping people deal with stress.

> A study of 44 women at University of Arkansas for Medical Sciences found that those who participated in a 12-week stress management-augmented behavioural weight loss intervention not only had lower cortisol (stress hormone) levels but they also lost more weight.[33]

Chapter 6: **Forgiveness**

'To err is human; to forgive divine.'
(Alexander Pope)

Resentment: A Weight on Your Shoulders

It should be no surprise that resentment related to negative childhood experiences is inextricably linked to your weight and/or binge eating. Research has confirmed that negative life experiences during childhood play a major role in the development of obesity, potentially by causing mental and emotional disturbances, poor coping responses, stress, inflammation, and metabolic disturbances.[1] A systematic review and analysis of 112,708 participants in the journal *Obesity Review* found that adults with reported childhood abuse were significantly more likely to be obese. All four types of abuse were significantly associated with adult obesity: physical, emotional, sexual, and general abuse. Severe abuse was significantly more associated with adult obesity compared with light/moderate abuse.

If you have been abused, you can probably relate to the findings how much abuse can interfere with your efforts to lose weight. Abuse in childhood, and even in adulthood, can be stressful. You may find it difficult to cope with daily stressors, including coping with hunger, cravings, and poor body image because it is impacted so much by the trauma of previous abuse.

If you have not experienced what is considered traumatic 'abuse', but you still feel like your past has been stressful, you are like many others. Trauma or abuse need not be in the form of physical hitting, sexual molestation, witnessing domestic violence, conventional emotional abuse, or emotional abandonment by a caretaker. I have had many patients who have witnessed their parents fighting and finding that traumatic; not being accepted by a step-parent; being neglected or rejected by a parent; not getting support or encouragement from a parent or teacher; being bullied by a sibling or classmate ... This list is, of course, not complete.

I have had patients in my office minimising these sorts of events, saying, 'I wasn't abused. I had a good childhood. I shouldn't feel like this ... other people have had it worse!' Yet, the important thing is not what happened or what did not happen. The important thing is the way you perceived and responded to it. There's no right or wrong way of responding to anything. You responded to something that was beyond your ability to cope.

Thus, whether you have experienced what is considered 'abuse' or have responded to something like abuse, the fact is that this abuse is not in the past. The event may not be happening anymore, but your response is continuing to traumatise you. If you are still responding to the past, it means that the trauma is still haunting you. One of the main ways trauma can affect you is resentment, which is a state of 'non-forgiveness'. Ask yourself, *Can I forgive ... for doing ... to me?* If your answer is no, it means the past is holding you back from moving forward, even letting go of excess weight or an eating problem.

This chapter is about letting go of that past so that you can let go of your fat and out of control eating.

Resentment is natural, normal, and understandable. Whether you are resenting someone who hurt you or whether it is something you think should no longer be upset about. I had a patient who came to see me for panic attacks. She outlined how she had them even as a fifteen-year-old teenager. One day it got so bad she was crying in her bedroom and couldn't go to school. Instead of being comforted by her parents, her mother told her, 'Don't be so silly,' and her father blamed her for upsetting her mother and being a bad example for her sister. This made her angry with her parents. To heal this resentment (as minor as it may seem), we needed to start out by allowing herself to feel angry and acknowledge that her parents didn't provide her with the support she needed. She had downplayed how ineffective her parents acted in this situation just as much as she downplayed her own feelings of anger towards them. She had always said, 'But they gave me a good childhood. I shouldn't be angry with them.'

Her parents did the best they could. They may not have intended to do any harm, but that's not the way it was perceived by her. Also, her parents aren't perfect. Even if they had done 99 percent correct parenting, 1 percent is still not perfect. Even 1 percent wrongdoing is still wrongdoing. Resentment about a single event like this (or even several little events like this) doesn't mean she needed to punish them. Neither is it a black-and-white situation of either resenting them totally or not resenting them at all. It was about allowing herself to feel resentment for that specific event while still loving them and forgiving them for their minor mistake.

Can you find a similar event in your past? Something that you find hard to forgive, yet you know the other person had the best intentions at heart? Using the above example, can you apply the same principles to forgive a person? The important aspect here though again is that: (1) It is okay to be angry and have resentment. (2) It is necessary to forgive to set yourself free of disordered eating and weight problems, (3) It is also okay *not* to reconcile with the perpetrator, even after you have forgiven him or her.

Abuse or trauma is anything that made you feel guilty, ashamed, helpless, hopeless, terrified, depressed, abandoned, enraged, anxious, or empty—whether it was a once-off or a repeated occurrence.

Abuse or trauma is anything that made you believe, 'I'm not good enough/inadequate, there's something wrong with me, I'm permanently damaged, I'm not in control, my body is hateful, I'm shameful, I did something wrong, I should have done something, I'm a failure, I can't succeed … ' etc.

Research has proven that resentment can be the cause of disease.[2] For example, investigators have proven that thoughts of revenge lead to cardiovascular and sympathetic nervous system arousal. More specifically, a study by Hope College has found that simply thinking about resentment not only causes negative emotions, but also a rise in blood pressure and heart rate.[3] It can be said that when people hold a grudge, they stay in the victim role and that nursing a grudge is considered a commitment to remain angry.[4]

Research has also shown that forgiveness can, in fact, enhance health[5] and can facilitate cardiovascular and sympathetic nervous system arousal to return to normal.[6] For weight management and control of eating, forgiveness appears to be pivotal. Since starting to work as a clinician, I worked a great deal with people who had been sexually abused. Nine times of ten, weight/fat was a problem. Many believed they had put the weight on to become unattractive to avoid another unwanted sexual experience. In other words, fat served as a form of protection. Others explained their binges as an escape from having to deal with the emotional pain of the memory/memories. Resentment and hatred was a major issue.

Patients who had come to me with the aim of freeing themselves from sexual trauma received great relief by working to release resentment. The side-effect of treatment was a relief in bingeing and loss of excess weight. I had several surprise phone calls from patients who told me about how their desire to overeat just somehow disappeared. I can demonstrate a particular example of a case of a forty-year-old patient who had struggled with her weight since age twelve. Her history was nothing overly remarkable, mild compared to other patients. There was no sexual abuse. She had an alcoholic mother who was an irresponsible parent, a father who was neglectful (due to long work hours and affairs), and a brother who bullied her. When we established that she resented all three of them for doing her harm, we identified that no diet would ever succeed as long as she felt resentful. She recognised that she sabotaged her weight loss by bingeing (especially on chocolate), being tempted to blow a diet every time she felt hopeless or saw or smelled her favourite food, and staying fat for twenty-eight years.

When I made her realise that she is continuing to let these three people torture her many years later, she said, 'Stuff all of them. Let me prove to them they no longer have power over me.' From then on, every time she had the thought of not being able to control her eating, she said, 'Stuff them!' That was her mantra. With that mantra in her head, she was able to limit her food intake, no longer had binges, and achieved her ideal weight. She said each time she had an overwhelming craving for food or chocolate, she just told herself, 'No, you (the perpetrator) can't win. I win this time!' She refused to let them beat her and won her battle of the bulge.

We Cannot Change Weight by Holding Onto Things That Created It

Forgiveness has been defined as the wilful giving up of resentment in the face of another's injustice and responding with beneficence to the offender, even though that offender has no right to the forgiver's moral goodness. Forgiveness is distinguished from *condoning, justification, excusing, reconciling*, and *forgetting*.

Forgiveness is not easy yet forgiveness is necessary. Business philosopher Jim Rohn said, 'you must take personal responsibility. You cannot change the circumstances, the seasons, or the wind, but you can change yourself.' Einstein too said, 'we cannot change a problem with the same things that created it.' Believing you can change your eating and your weight while still resenting is virtually impossible. The thing about blame is that:

No matter how much you blame someone, it will not give you what you want. It simply keeps you at the same place you were when you were victimised. You can't change what happened, but you can change how you feel about what happened. Nothing changes until you change.

I have seen other such transformations when forgiveness takes place and personal responsibility steps in that place. The beauty of forgiveness is that it's something that you can do. You're never stuck with having to resent someone. Just like the world famous magician Dynamo: he experienced bullying—a very negative experience. Instead of being the victim and feeling sorry for himself, he is now a famous world-class magician making millions for *a skill he gained because he was bullied*. For more information, go to Dynamo's website.

In conventional psychotherapy, forgiveness exercises—amongst other things—involve writing a letter to the perpetrator, telling him or her how you feel, how much you're hurting, etc. The writer of the letter is told to burn rather than send the letter. This may or may not work for you. Find out what works for you. If you have experienced a sexual trauma, I would recommend going to psychological therapy. EMDR (explained in a later chapter) is a treatment that—in my clinical experience—is best at facilitating trauma. You may also find the 'Hyp2HipSlimming' DVD Troubleshooting section helpful.

'Our challenges are not supposed to paralyse us; they're supposed to help us discover who we really are.' (Bernice Johnson Reagon)

If you are in a situation in which you cannot forgive yourself for something and believe you don't deserve to be happy, remember Buddha's advice: 'you yourself, as much as anybody in the entire universe, deserve your love and affection.' One of my patients attended therapy with me because she was told by her employer to attend. Apart from depressed mood, she lacked energy, was 15kg overweight, was irritable (with her grandchildren, colleagues, and children), and avoided social interaction including parties and other functions. She was non-compliant with her anti-depressant medication and seemed reluctant to engage in therapy. When I asked why she did not want to get better, she said, 'I've done such horrible things. I don't deserve to be better.' When we addressed those 'horrible things' she had done, she became a different person—her energy improved, she had asked me to assist her to lose weight, and her colleagues commented on how pleasant she was to be around.

A prime example of how resentment can hold you back is of a patient who came to me because he was depressed. Upon assessment, we discovered sexual abuse. He stated that this had impacted his entire life: his confusion about his sexuality (which developed into a sex addiction), his career choice, his self-esteem, his ability to have relationships (of which several fell apart). He was in the process of legal proceedings regarding his abuse and was waiting for compensation payment. I asked how the payment would make him feel, he responded by saying it would ease his financial worries. While he was waiting for this payment, he sustained a work injury and ended up walking with a cane. He wanted workers compensation and waited for this too. He had waited for 6 months and in the meantime his depression deteriorated and his weight increased. Unfortunately, I don't know if he did eventually receive the compensation as I had recognised he did not want to get better (improve his depression) and stopped seeing him. He was focused on getting financial compensation, not focused on improving his mental and physical health.

'The weak can never forgive. Forgiveness is the attribute of the strong.' (Mahatma Gandhi)

10 Guidelines to Understand Forgiveness

Many of my patients have not wanted to forgive their perpetrators, believing that doing so would endorse their behaviour. Rest assured. I will not advise you to say to your perpetrators 'what you did was okay' or 'what you did does not matter.' Instead, I will ask you to consider how resentment has served you. Has it been helpful or hurtful. For example, if a friend came to visit you and broke one of your favourite cups by accident, would you initially be angry but then evaluate: 'is my cup worth more than the friendship?' The following guidelines should help you lighten your load.

'Holding anger is a poison. It eats you from inside. We think that hating is a weapon that attacks the person who harmed us. But hatred is a curved blade. And the harm we do, we do to ourselves.' (Mitch Albom, The Five People You Meet in Heaven)

1. Release anger and reclaim your power

If you were to look at how the perpetrator changed your life, identify if the change is for the better. If you are unable to identify how the perpetrator has improved your life, evaluate whether holding onto resentment is going to serve you. Think of forgiveness as a gift you can give yourself. In forgiving, ask yourself: 'who wins? The perpetrator or me?' If the answer is that the perpetrator wins, is it time to forgive? According to philosopher Neblett, 'the essence of forgiveness is in the decision to forgive, along with the proclamation 'I forgive you'.' Best of all: you do not have to say it to the perpetrator directly.

> *'Always forgive your enemies - nothing annoys them so much.'* (Oscar Wilde)

2. Gain insight to lose the fat

Observe the world around you: do bad things happen to good people? Is the world fair? Does the way people behave always make sense? If you were to understand why the perpetrator acted the way he or she did, would that help you? For example, a parent who has hurt you, may refuse to admit this or apologise or make up for it as he or she may be too proud, too narcissistic, or too ashamed. Some perpetrators may fear legal repercussions or not being able to engage in their addiction.

> *'To forgive is the highest, most beautiful form of love. In return, you will receive untold peace and happiness.'* (Robert Muller)

3. Rise above victimhood to lower your weight

Identify whether holding onto resentment has led to any changes. When you think of the event, are you still the victim even after all this time? If you want to no longer be the victim, change how you think about it. The worst part of the resistance to healing doesn't come from what actually happened in the past, but long after the event, the ongoing story about it, and the shadows it continues to cast in your life.

> *'To forgive is to set a prisoner free and discover that the prisoner was you.'* (Lewis B. Smedes)

4. Do not be the one to cast the first stone

Acknowledge that you have also perpetrated in your life and needed someone's forgiveness too.

5. Trust that the perpetrator will be punished

If you were to look at all those people who wronged you, do you believe they will be punished for their wrongdoings? Do you trust that the universe will punish the perpetrator more than you or any court ruling could ever do? Do you believe that there is such a thing as karma? If not, how can you reconcile with the fact that the world really is not fair and that bad people get away with bad stuff?

6. Exclude any revenge tactics

Catherine Ponder said, 'When you hold resentment toward another, you are bound to that person or condition by an emotional link that is stronger than steel. Forgiveness is the only way to dissolve that link and get free.' Remember too that any motivation to hurt the one who has hurt you means that you have the capacity for harm. Is that who you are too? Are you just as bad as the perpetrator?

'Forgiveness has nothing to with absolving a criminal of his crime. It has everything to do with relieving oneself of the burden of being a victim—letting go of the pain and transforming oneself from victim to survivor.' (C.R.Straham)

7. Accept it was meant to be

It may seem very odd to say that something horrible happened to you for a reason. But why else did it happen? What happened is guiding you to your purpose. I had a patient who resented her father for leaving the family and not providing any financial support. Once she recognised that it was the reason she had so much energy to provide for her own family, she released resentment and was even grateful for being in that situation. Jack Canfield, a prolific author of many books including the *Chicken Soup* series, said of forgiveness, 'being negative, angry, and unforgiving about a past hurt only ensures that you will attract more of the same into your life. You can choose to stay stuck in victimhood or choose to be a survivor and transcend that experience and be better off because you have had the experience.'

8. Turn the trauma into a positive

If resentment had the power to hurt that person, to erase what happened to you, to make you better off, to heal your pain, then continue resenting all you want. Has it? Or has resentment done nothing except hurt you even more? An example of how a trauma has been turned into a positive is the story of how the organisation MADD (Mother Against Drunk Drivers) started. It began with a parent losing a child due to being killed by a drunk driver. She could have chosen to live in resentment towards this drunk driver all her life. Instead, she started MADD, which implemented Alcohol Breath Testing Stations across roads in South Africa.

Another example of how resentment has served a purpose was that of Dave Pelzer. He is the author of several books including *The Child Called It, The Lost Boy,* and *A Man Named Dave*. I said it's an example of how he benefitted from resentment only because he benefitted in three ways: he made more than enough money from selling his books to buy his dream house in his favourite location, he met his wife through writing his books (she was in the publishing business), and he was responsible for changing some foster care laws!

My own story of how I found my path to writing this book (as outlined in the preface) is similar. I had several perpetrators in my life who I could have chosen not to forgive. But what purpose did that serve? Instead, I chose to turn that tragic situation into something I would find meaning in—I found my calling (as a psychologist), was driven to achieve my own weight management goal, and am making money from it! It's a win situation for me and continues to be a lose situation for my perpetrators! I've had a few patients change their career path due to their transformation—one patient told me she was going back to university to focus her research on bullying at school and come up with a preventative program. Another decided to become a fitness instructor at age fifty-six!

So, to answer this question: 'how have you benefitted from your traumatic event?' think of how you can benefit from your 'tragedy.' Whether it's doing something big like writing your book about what happened (like Dave Pelzer), starting an organisation to stop the same happening to other people (like MADD), finding your career path, becoming an educator at school about 'stranger danger' ... the possibilities are endless and your passion about this can be too.

> *'Resentment is like drinking poison and then hoping it will kill your enemies.* (Nelson Mandela, former president of South Africa and Nobel Peace Prize winner)

9. Forgive but never forget

Thomas S. Szasz said, 'The stupid neither forgive nor forget; the naive forgive and forget; the wise forgive but do not forget.' It's unlikely that you can ever forget events that have shaped you for so long and in so many ways. But forgiveness is a different thing.

10. Accept that compensation for the trauma is not possible

I have had various patients over the years who have gone to court due to wanting to convict their rapist or abuser or get worker's compensation for the trauma they suffered. But how does a conviction or money ever make up for what happened? If you were to come up with a figure (financially) how much would you like? Would that make up for it? How do you expect the perpetrator to make it up to you? If you would be satisfied with a court conviction or a financial compensation, go for it. For me—in my situation—I decided there was no amount of money or apologies that the perpetrators in my life could compensate for what they had done to me. I realised I had to move on. Can you? Do you have another choice that will set you free? Remember that forgiveness does not depend on whether the perpetrator ever acknowledges the harm(s) he or she caused you.

Exercises to Release Resentment to Release the Fat

Exercise 1: Write down why you think you're fat or have eating problems in terms of possible emotional trauma in the past. Whether these are serious ones (e.g. sexual abuse) or comparatively minor ones (e.g. being told by mom, 'You're not good enough') Who do you resent? What do you feel sad about? Who do you envy? What irritates you? Your task today is to identify who hurt you, feel the anger, and identify what the consequences of your resentment are. Identify how much better off you are for having had that experience and forgive—stop the war on yourself.

Exercise 2: Go online to read about 'The Forgiveness Project' and Gill Hicks' incredible story of surviving the 2005 train bomb in London, or read some excellent tips on forgiveness—for example, a very short but very good booklet *Forgiveness Therapy* by David Shell (Abbey Press). Alternatively, read one of Dave Pelzer's books.

Exercise 3: Answer the question: how can I benefit from my trauma?

Exercise 4: Watch the 'Hyp2Hip Slimming DVD', specifically the 'Troubleshooting' section

Chapter 7: **Sleep Away Your Fat**

'My doctor told me to stop having intimate dinners for four – unless there are three other people.'
(Orson Welles)

Imagine waking up one morning and being the shape and size you want to be ... imagine that it could be facilitated just by sleeping better ... *Weight Off Your Mind* is here to tell you that you can dream through your sleep but not sleep through your dream to achieve your weight management goal.

A study at the University of Wisconsin Medical School found that reduced sleep makes you feel hungrier because of reduced leptin and elevated ghrelin levels[1]

Wake Up to Your Best Body

It turns out when you wake up makes a difference to your weight. About 20 minutes of sunlight assists in producing a sleep hormone (melatonin) and synchronising your body rhythm, which helps you sleep better. However, getting more sunshine can also help you lose weight—according to a study from Northwestern University Feinberg School of

Medicine.[2] Researchers tracked fifty-four participants' exposure to morning light with a wrist monitor for seven days. They discovered that those who got more morning light had lower BMIs than those who got less—and that was regardless of their age, how active they were, and what they ate. It appears that exposing yourself to light early in the morning as opposed to later in the day synchronises your internal body clock, which means that you are more likely to have a natural and steady sleep schedule. In turn, that steady sleep schedule helps your metabolism run more efficiently.

Morning light (which has a higher amount of blue light) is much stronger than afternoon or evening light and thus has the strongest effect on your circadian rhythm. It doesn't take much—as little as 20–30 minutes of morning sunlight between 8 a.m. and noon. Of course, while you need to protect yourself from the sun with sunscreen to avoid skin cancer, direct sun exposure is also necessary for your Vitamin D requirements. The importance of sleep was further highlighted by a study on melatonin in the Breakthrough Generations Study.[3] This study of 100,000 women over nine years found that those who were exposed to light at night had greater incidences of obesity than those who did not.

Sleep Away Your Fat Tip 1

Expose yourself to at least 20 minutes of morning light and be sure to get good quality sleep in the dark at night.

Better Sleep for Reduced Hunger

If you think that you can afford the luxury of staying up all night to watch TV or stay on the internet, then here are a few facts that will jolt you back into taking care of your body by providing it with sufficient sleep. Research has proven that:

- Even a single night of sleep deprivation increases ghrelin levels which increases feelings of hunger[4]
- Sleep deprivation leads to increased cortisol levels (the stress hormone which inhibits weight loss)[5]
- When people are sleep deprived (even four hours less), they consume 22 percent more (559 +/- 617 calories) and are hungrier before breakfast and dinner[6]

Apart from being associated with several chronic diseases, sleep restriction is associated with:

- Changes in leptin levels (the hormone that makes you feel satiated)
- Changes in ghrelin levels (the hormones that makes you feel hungry)
- Changes in orexin/hypocretin levels (the hormones responsible for appetite)
- Changes in glucose metabolism (how your body processes sugar)
- Changes in your autonomic nervous system (the part that controls bodily functions, including your heartbeat and digestive processes)

All of the above lead to increased food intake and preference for energy-dense foods and weight gain and a higher obesity risk in the long-term.[7]

Sufficient and good quality sleep decreases your hunger hormones and helps muscles recover, which leads to a healthy metabolism.

If you are finding excuses for not getting enough sleep, ensure that you address these whether it is watching too much television or spending too much time on Facebook or other computer activities. If you are a mother of young children who disturb your sleep, I understand that this is a problem that is not simple to solve. I've had several patients in my office who are mothers of newborns complaining of poor quality sleep due to baby waking them several times at night. First the nightly feeds, then the teething, then the constant desire of the toddler to sleep with you. You may be surprised how this seemingly incurable problem can be solved. One particular patient I had, for example, was a young mother who stated that she hadn't slept well for the past three years since the birth of her baby. I suggested she speak to a paediatric nurse. A week later, she reported that the solution was simple—simpler than expected. She set boundaries with her toddler to sleep in her own bed and while it was not easy the first few nights, once done, she had a wonderful night's sleep and ever since! If you have a baby or young kids who disrupt your sleep, at the very least attempt to alleviate some of problem by discussing it with a paediatrician or paediatric nurse. I spoke to a paediatric nurse who said a baby should be able to sleep through the night from as early as three months old, but six months old is more common. If at twelve months your baby is not sleeping through the night, this may indicate a problem that you can certainly discuss with your paediatrician. Most of it is probably normal, but you may be surprised what can be done. I'm not saying it's easy in all cases, but at least try to solve it rather than assuming it cannot be solved.

Sleep Away the Fat Tip 2:

Melt your fat and curb your eating by ensuring you get enough sleep.

If you already sleep well, keep going with your good sleep habits. If you don't sleep well, read the following:

How to Get Better Sleep (Even if You Have Young Children)

Temporary insomnia can be caused by worry or stress about work or other stressors. Should the insomnia occur at least three times per week for more than a month and causes you significant distress, it is considered a disorder. Insomnia is symptomised by difficulty falling asleep, difficulty staying asleep, or early morning waking or restlessness.[8]

Insomnia can be caused by a variety of things. In my clinical experience, it is mostly due to a mood disorder (e.g. depression) and anxiety. If it's depression, find solutions in the chapter on depression. I've had several patients who also struggle with sleep due to medication side effects or medical conditions such as sleep apnoea, diabetes, and pain. In some cases, insomnia is simply due to poor sleep habits or shift work that disrupts the body's natural ability to sleep. One of my patients discovered that by eliminating the foods she was sensitive to, she was able to sleep much better. Another patient told me once she had gone to her dietitian (who had recommended magnesium supplementation), she slept much better. I've had several people who had great improvements in their quality of sleep after tart cherry or melatonin. If you're struggling with sleep, go to: www.https/

sleepfoundation.org or www.https/helpguide.org and find help to sleep better.

If you have chronic sleep problems, you have several options. Conventional sleeping pills 'benzodiazepines' (e.g. Temazepam, Stilnox) should be your last resort as they are addictive and have other negative side effects including memory loss. Your GP may be able to prescribe alternative medications such as Zyprexa or Seroquel, although even milder ones like anti-histamines may be sufficient. If you are depressed, your GP is more likely to prescribe an anti-depressant (e.g. Desyrel, Elavil, Mirtazapine) which may assist with sleep. Topiramate—a medication that has actually been found to be effective for weight loss[9], has also been effective for night eating syndrome.[10]

As a first line intervention, try the following:[11]

- Keep a regular sleep schedule. This is the simplest, cheapest and most effective way to eliminate insomnia. Go to sleep at the same time every night and wake up at the same time every morning. Doing this will take discipline but will significantly reduce risk of having a tough time sleeping. For example, go to bed and sleep 10 p.m. to 6 a.m., regardless of dinner parties, TV shows, weekends, etc. Once awake, get out of bed! Do not lie in bed.
- The most difficult part of getting into a regular sleep schedule is the first 2 weeks—after that your body will become accustomed to it and your body will automatically slot into this routine; avoid naps at all costs! If initially you can't fall asleep, get out of bed and engage in a relaxing activity (e.g. reading) rather than lie in bed awake. You can start this ritual by forcing yourself out of bed at 6 a.m. and staying awake until 10 p.m.

- Have a bedtime ritual. Your body will learn to associate certain activities with 'time to sleep.' This may include having a warm bath, reading a book, listening to a relaxation tape, sexual activity, doing progressive muscle relaxation, or watching TV (nothing too stimulating/exciting or thought-provoking). Hypnotise yourself by taking three deep, slow breaths and repeat three times, 'Go to sleep now,' when you are ready to fall asleep.
- Eat a healthy diet. Eating a heavy meal for dinner leads to increased blood flow for a few hours that, for some people, can cause too much stimulation for sleep. Although some naturopaths believe that certain foods can stimulate serotonin/tryptophan production and thus make you sleepy (cheese, turkey, milk, banana, etc.), this theory has not been proven. But you could try. A few health websites say that certain foods can be stimulating i.e. spicy, rich, or heavy foods; cayenne pepper; food additives; pork; eggplant; dairy; wheat; corn; chocolate; and spinach. However, this theory hasn't been proven sufficiently either.
- Avoid caffeinated products including coffee, Coke, V, Red Bull, tea, chocolate, and other stimulants including guarana, ephedrine (still found in some 'flu remedies'), green tea, kola nut, and ginseng.
- Avoid alcohol. Whereas alcohol can assist sleep onset, it can cause disturbed sleep patterns. Because of their opposing actions and different half-lives (amount of time it takes to metabolise in the body), alcohol and caffeine taken together can produce insomnia as it causes a rebound effect.[12]
- Exercise daily. Apart from other benefits, exercise reduces physical stress on the body and assists the body to sleep. At least 30 minutes of aerobic exercise

is recommended (e.g. walking, swimming, jogging). Avoid exercising immediately before bedtime.

- Practice progressive muscle relaxation or listen to a relaxation CD while lying in bed (see the chapter on stress management for further information).
- Have a relaxed attitude about sleep. Don't worry if you can't sleep as you would like. Think about it, the worst possible result if you don't sleep well or not long enough is that you'll feel tired—this is not fatal, just very unpleasant. Also keep in mind that while most adults need eight hours of sleep, you may need less. If you don't fall asleep within 30 minutes, get up, go to another room, and do something not too arousing. Avoid clock watching. If you continue to worry about sleep, the worry will keep you awake.
- Keep a sleep diary to track your sleep (instead of making assumptions), track your sleep for two weeks. A Fitbit or similar device can assist.
- Manage anxiety and depression. Practice coping skills (e.g. positive self-talk) and engage in social activities and hobbies to avoid worrying and being depressed about things. If anxiety and depression are persistent and interfere with your normal functioning, seek help from a psychologist.
- Avoid any disruptions. Don't let a pet or child sleep in your room if this causes your sleep to be disturbed. If you have a partner who snores, make sure to get this problem eliminated. It could just be a matter of going to the pharmacy to get a nasal strip, sleeping in separate bedrooms, or as much as having to get a C-Pap machine to manage sleep apnoea.
- Make your sleeping environment conducive to sleep:

- Ensure your room is a comfortably temperature—warm, not too hot/cold.
- Ensure the room is quiet—no music, noisy neighbours, no TV. Wear earplugs if necessary.
- Have a relaxing, dark environment—no stimulating coloured red/orange/pink curtains, rather have dark blue/dark green curtains; no bright lights.
- Keep the room fresh—aired, clean, non-polluted, not breezy.
- Ensure the mattress is comfortable and less than ten years old.
- Use your bed only for sleep and sex. Never ever eat in bed (not even breakfast in bed).

Sleep Your Fat Away Quick Guide:

✓ If you have diabetes or pain that is preventing you from sleeping well, address this (e.g. by going to speak to your GP)

✓ If you feel tired during the day and/or your partner notices that you snore heavily, speak to your GP to check if it's sleep apnoea

✓ If your sleep has not been good since starting a medication, speak to your pharmacist or GP about an alternative and/or how to deal with the side-effects

✓ If you're depressed, read the chapter on depression

✓ If you're anxious, use the methods in the stress management chapter to help you sleep better

✓ Get into a good sleep routine and ensure your sleep environment is conducive to sleep

✓ As much as possible, eliminate the causes of sleep disruptions (I don't mean you need to get rid of your children!).

Part III

Psych Check: How to Make Hypnosis Work by Removing Psychological Barriers

Chapter 8: **Get in the Mood for Weight Management**

'The pessimist complains about the wind; the optimist expects it to change; the realist adjusts the sails.'
(William A Ward)

Are you depressed because you lose control over your eating, can't stop gaining weight, hate what your body looks like? Or do you lose control over eating, fail to stop weight gain, hate your body because you're depressed? If you find yourself craving and eating chocolate, carbohydrates, or any food to lift your mood, this chapter aims to provide you with information about what depression is and how to lift yourself out of it so that you no longer eat to cope with it. This would apply whether you have a full blown depressive disorder or simply have mood dips.

Mood Up, Weight Down: How Your Mood May be Linked to Your Eating and Weight

If you tend to have carbohydrate cravings, especially when you are feeling depressed, you may be able to relate to the findings in a study conducted at the University of Alabama: researchers discovered that those who craved carbohydrates felt distressed prior to their cravings and satisfied, happy, and relaxed after eating carbohydrates. Those who craved protein reported feeling anxious or hungry prior to their cravings and happy, normal, bored, and energetic after eating protein-rich food. The researchers found that intense mood states lead to cravings, especially cravings for sweet carbohydrates.[1] Another study of 931 adults found those who were depressed also ate more chocolate (8.4 servings per month) compared to non-depressed people (5.4 servings per month). Those with the highest scores of depression also had the highest chocolate consumption (11.8 servings per month).[2]

If you tend to crave chocolate when you are depressed, you may also be able to identify with the findings in a study conducted at the University of Wuerzburg in Germany: the researchers concluded that eating tasty chocolate immediately lifted negative mood for three minutes. The researchers believe that it's because of this immediate mood lift (even if it's so temporary), that chocolate-eating becomes a habitual way to cope with stress.[3]

Research has confirmed that those who lose weight and maintain weight loss are less likely to be depressed.[4]

In my practice I have seen how prevalent the combination of Binge Eating Disorder is with the mood disorder, commonly referred to as 'depression'. In psychology we call it 'comborbidity' (when two or more disorders co-occur). This isn't necessarily a bad thing, as I have seen many times how eliminating one disorder has a knock-on effect on the other disorder. For example, a patient who came to me for treatment—referred by her psychiatrist—said she was there to address her 'depression'. She weighed 135 kg at 170 cm. Asked whether she was depressed about her weight, she said, 'I suppose …' but couldn't identify a specific trigger for her depression. When I suggested working on reducing her weight/binge eating, she agreed to do so. Once she started losing weight and being more in control of her eating, the depression also lifted and her suicidal ideation became a thing of the past. I personally found that my premenstrual symptoms disappeared once I lost 12kg (72kg to 60kg). Premenstrual discomfort—in my opinion—should not be the norm. Neither should it be endured, in the belief that it's just a normal part of being a woman.

What this means for you is you may find that when you heal your eating/weight, your depression (and possibly also premenstrual symptoms) may lift too. Or, once you treat your depression and premenstrual discomfort, your weight/eating issues may be resolved too. The reason it's important to clear your depression is because research has proven:[5]

- Patients with depression only attained 63 percent of the weight loss compared to non-depressed patients
- Only 27 percent of patients with both depression and a Binge Eating Disorder achieved clinically significant weight loss compared with 67 percent of patients who had neither disorder

Research has confirmed that obesity (particularly abdominal obesity) is associated with major depressive disorder.[6]

Depression Defined

What exactly is 'depression?' Occasional depressed mood differs from actual mood disorder in that a disorder is associated with many other symptoms in addition to depressed mood. For example, most people who have major depressive disorder also have either lack of appetite and weight loss or increased appetite and weight gain. Apart from appetite/food cravings and weight, there are many other symptoms of depression, depending on which type of depression it is. Go through the following checklists to check.

Major Depressive Disorder Checklist Check 'yes' if you have had the following symptoms regularly for at least 2 weeks and they are affecting your ability to function at home or work	Check if yes
1. I feel depressed most of the time (sad, empty, hopeless, with or without crying; or irritable)	
2. I am unable to enjoy things	
Continue only if you have checked yes to either 1 or 2.	
3. I sleep either too much or too little (or have interrupted sleep)	
4. My weight and appetite is either too high (or too low)	
5. I feel lethargic most of the time	
6. I feel either agitated, restless, or slowed down	
7. I have frequent feelings of guilt and/or worthlessness	

8. I struggle a great deal with memory and/or concentration	
9. I have suicidal thoughts, sometimes as far as having a plan and intention to go ahead with a suicide or just thoughts of not wanting to be around*	

**If you have suicidal thoughts, please seek help from your GP and a psychologist immediately and contact a crisis helpline. Call Lifeline on 13 11 14*

If you have checked yes to at least 5 of questions 3 to 9 and feel significantly affected by these symptoms and have them despite not taking a drug or having a medical condition, you may have major depressive disorder (MDD). This is not meant as a diagnostic test. It is a guideline only, based on the Diagnostic and Statistical Manual (DSM-5).7 Only a qualified mental health care professional (psychologist, psychiatrist) can diagnose.

Another milder version of the above type of depression is called Adjustment Disorder (with depressed features). You may also be familiar with post-natal depression, which occurs after giving birth. Bipolar Affective Disorder (B.A.D.), on the other hand, is another type of mood disorder in which periods of depression alternate with several weeks or months of mania. Symptoms of mania include feeling ecstatic, grandiose, needing less sleep, feeling pressure to keep talking, having racing thoughts, excessive energy, and irritability. B.A.D. also affects appetite and weight but usually involves poor appetite.

'When the heart weeps for what it has lost, the spirit laughs at what is has gained.' (Sufi proverb)

Seasonal Affective Disorder (S.A.D.) Checklist Check 'yes' if you have had the following symptoms more so in colder winter months	Check if yes
I eat more and crave carbohydrates such as bread and pasta	
I have gained weight	
I feel sad, grumpy, moody, or anxious	
I have lost interest in my usual activities	
I sleep more and feel drowsy during the daytime	

If you have any of the above symptoms and have them despite not taking a drug or having a medical condition, you may have Seasonal Affective Disorder (SAD).[7] This is a guideline only, not a diagnostic test. Only a qualified mental health care professional (psychologist, psychiatrist) can diagnose.

Persistent Depressive Disorder (Formerly Dysthymic Disorder) **Checklist** Check 'yes' if you have experienced the following symptoms regularly for at least two years and find that your ability to function properly at home/work is affected	Check if yes
I overeat regularly	
I have sleep disturbance (especially sleeping too much)	
I feel fatigued a great deal	
I have poor self-esteem	
I have difficulty concentrating and making decisions	
I feel hopeless a great deal of the time	
I feel depressed (or irritable) a great deal	

If you have checked at least 2 of the above symptoms, and have them despite not taking a drug or have a medical condition, you may Persistent Depressive Disorder.[7] This is a guideline only, not meant as a diagnostic test. Only a qualified mental health care professional (psychologist, psychiatrist) can diagnose.

Pre-Menstrual Dysphoric Disorder (PMDD)[7] Checklist—for women only Check 'yes' if you have at least 5 of the following symptoms about 5-7 days before most menstrual cycles most of the year:	Check if yes
I feel depressed, hopeless, or have self-deprecating thoughts	
I feel anxious or tense	
I feel very sensitive, e.g. suddenly feeling sad or tearful	
I feel angry a great deal or am irritable and have more arguments with loved ones	
I have lost interest and enjoyment in activities	
I have difficulty concentrating	
I feel lethargic	
I crave food and overeat a great deal	
My sleep is disrupted: I have hypersomnia or insomnia	
I feel overwhelmed	
I have physical symptoms i.e., breast tenderness, headaches, joint or muscle pain, bloating, water retention/weight gain, swelling acne, gastrointestinal disturbances, dizziness or other pain incl. dysmenorrhea (cramps/ 'period pain')	

These symptoms may increase with puberty, 1-2 years prior to menopause, upon discontinuing oral contraceptives, or occur due to pregnancy complicated by toxemia, or after a period of amenorrhea, or after tubal ligation, psychological stress or trauma. To diagnose correctly, women are advised to keep a diary to note symptoms. This is a guideline only, not a diagnostic test. Only a qualified health care professional can diagnose.

Many people with above mentioned depressive disorders also complain of having headaches or greater pain sensitivity and sexual dysfunctions. Alternative health professionals sometimes refer to the above disorders as a 'serotonin deficiency syndrome'.

Causes of Depression

There is a strong genetic link with depression—if one or both of your parents have depression, you are more likely to have depression yourself.[8] However, your environment can also trigger depression. It should be no surprise that depressive disorders can also be brought on by childhood trauma, e.g. sexual abuse, but also recent stress like divorce, poor social support, work stress, etc.[9] But you may be surprised to learn that:

Dieting reduces tryptophan (the amino acid that produces the feel good chemical serotonin).[10]

Hence, the more you diet, the greater your risk of being depressed. It can really then turn into a vicious cycle: you are depressed because you can't stop eating and are fat, and you can't stop eating because you are depressed. If you're a woman, you are at increased risk of depression anyway as serotonin levels are lower in women.[11] Since carbohydrates (and not protein) act on the release of the feel-good brain chemical serotonin, people tend to crave carbohydrates to feel good or better. In effect, eating carbohydrates is a way of self-medicating the serotonin deficit.[12]

Researchers at the Department of Applied Biological Sciences and Clinical Research Center in Massachusetts have found that eating carbohydrate-rich foods is a way a person self-medicates low serotonin levels.[13]

It's this drug-like effect of carbohydrates that makes people want to indulge in carbohydrates. The desire for carbohydrates unfortunately does not only apply to a need to boost mood, it also seems to apply to anxiety—research has found that carbohydrate-rich lunches induce relaxation in men and drowsiness in women.[14] Similarly, Stanford University researchers found that when people are in a negative mood, they tend to have more loss of control over eating and more fat intake. They also have reductions in anxiety after eating.[15]

The reason that you're more likely to crave and/or binge in the late afternoon or after dinner is because serotonin levels are naturally lower by mid-afternoon and into the evening.[16]

The fact that anti-depressants—particularly SSRIs, which act on the feel good chemical serotonin—reduce carbohydrate cravings also proves that your body is simply trying to alert you to boost its serotonin levels.[17] Whereas it's normal to feel depressed occasionally, it's abnormal and problematic to eat to cope with depressed mood or actual Mood Disorder symptoms, especially if it becomes a habit. Fortunately, alternative ways to boost serotonin are available and you will be surprised how much of a breakthrough you will experience once you take more appropriate actions to raise your serotonin.

Your sweet cravings may be due to low serotonin levels. Hence, you eat sweets to lift depressed mood.

How to Conquer Depression

Your body may have figured out that it can naturally elevate serotonin levels, i.e. your mood, by eating lots of carbohydrates! While we want to applaud your body for listening to your needs, we want to introduce it to some alternatives that will also fulfil your desire to curb binge eating and achieve a slimmer body. You have at least six different options to conquer your depression:

Option 1: Anti-depressants

You may be familiar with anti-depressants such as Prozac. Whereas this medical option is not the only one, anti-depressants are certainly a good option if you have a full blown clinical mood disorder. The research generally supports the use of anti-depressants for the treatment of depressive disorders.[18] In a meta-analysis of 31 studies of more than 4,000 patients, researchers found that 41 percent of patients who were switched to placebo, relapsed, compared to 18 percent who remained on an anti-depressant.[19]

When I lived in the USA during the mid-1990s, Prozac was used by many people to lose weight. In fact, studies have found Prozac to be effective for weight loss! For example, in a study with 45 participants on fluoxetine (Prozac), participants lost 12kg and only regained 4kg.[20] However, I have met people who complained about side effects as the dose (usually 60mg) is about three times the dose needed to treat depression. Unfortunately, studies have found that Prozac tends to lose its weight loss power after six months.[21]

Prozac has also been used in the treatment of premenstrual dysphoria and has been found to be effective.[22] Oral contraceptives (e.g. Yaz or Yasmin) have also proven to be an effective treatment for premenstrual symptoms.[23] If you would like to consider anti-depressants, there are a few things to keep in mind:

Negative side effects: These vary depending on the type of anti-depressants. Most SSRIs (one type of anti-depressants) have side effects that may include insomnia, headaches, nausea, diarrhoea, loss of sex drive, runny nose, and sweating.[24] If you know people who have been on an anti-depressants, you may know that some people experience such unpleasant side-effects that they discontinue them altogether. If you experience these or don't feel any better after 3-6 weeks, ask your GP and/or your pharmacist what to do. The good news is that some people don't have any side-effects at all and some have them only mildly and/or temporarily. Do not assume that you will have unpleasant side-effects—you may or may not have any of them or may have them only for a few weeks.

One of the most important things to keep in mind when you go to a GP to get a prescription for an anti-depressant is to ensure that the ones they are prescribing are not those that cause an increase in appetite and/or weight gain. Some anti-depressants are notorious for weight/appetite increases. You need to be on the anti-depressant that either has no effect on appetite/weight and or even facilitates weight loss in addition to relieving depression (see the information in the body check chapter 'Dr to the Rescue.' If you're not careful, it can become even more complicated if you are taking medication for obesity-related medical conditions.[25]

In the early 1990s when I was depressed, I took Efexor (venlafaxine) which made me feel even worse. Years later I was put on Wellbutrin (bupropion) which made me feel better instantly without any negative side-effects. I cannot guarantee that anti-depressants will work for you, but I can say that in many years in clinical practice, I have seen the benefits in many of my patients, particularly in combination with psychological treatment. If you find that your GP is not knowledgeable enough to assist you, ask for a referral to a psychiatrist or go to another GP.

How long to stay on an anti-depressant: Whether you will benefit at all, a little bit, or entirely is hard to predict. But before you give up, thinking they just don't work, remember that anti-depressants will take a while to relieve your symptoms. Pharmacists usually say it takes 3-6 weeks. Your depression didn't come on instantly either, so be patient. Some people find that they feel much improved only after six weeks whereas others find it initially makes them feel better but then the effect peters out. If you think about discontinuing because you can't tolerate unpleasant side effects or because you feel like you aren't benefitting, talk to your prescriber about trying a different anti-depressant. There are so many different ones available. It may take a trial of several different ones until you find one that is right for you or you may be lucky and find the right one for you first time around.

Also, ensure you follow the prescriber's advice in regards to how long to stay on the anti-depressant. Do not be tempted to discontinue without consulting your prescriber first. The amount of time you need to be on it can vary from six months to two years or more. Ensure that you have resolved the trigger and taper off them according to your prescriber's recommendation. Don't discontinue because you feel better. It may take a few months to reduce the dose first prior to discontinuing.

Whereas anti-depressants can lift you out of the depression, they won't necessarily prevent you from relapsing. In other words, serotonin-based medications are only effective as long you are taking them.[26] To keep depression at bay, it's important to get psychological therapy for the things that triggered the depression in the first place.

Option 2: Psychological therapy

I have listed anti-depressants as option 1, although I don't necessarily mean it should be your first or only option. In fact, the research supports the combination of anti-depressants and psychological therapy in the treatment of depressive disorders.[27] However, even psychotherapy by itself can effectively treat depressive disorders. Unlike anti-depressants, cognitive behavior therapy (CBT) has also been shown to prevent relapse.[28] A study published in the *Archives of General Psychiatry* showed that those treated with cognitive therapy (either alone or in combination with medication) had less than half the relapse rate compared to patients in the medication only group.[29] It appears that providing cognitive therapy during acute treatment prevents relapse.

If you have a depressive disorder, I would highly recommend psychological therapy. Your psychologist and GP will identify whether you are suitable for anti-depressant if you are interested in going with that combination option. I've seen many patients in treatment improving a great deal with therapy only. In some cases, particularly if fatigue and poor concentrations interfere with the process in therapy, the addition of anti-depressant is warranted.

Option 3: Nutritional intervention

Naturopaths recommend eating tryptophan-enhancing foods including turkey, chicken, apples, blueberries, and sunflower seeds to beat depression. However, there is very little scientific evidence to support this recommendation. However, supplementation with l-tryptophan has received some support.[30] Several other amino acids including tyrosine, phenylalanine, and methionine have also been mentioned.

Supplementation with the vitamin B folate has received some scientific support,[31] but not enough to be recommended as a stand-alone treatment.[32] Interestingly, research published in the *British Journal of Nutrition* stated that eating folate/folic acid rich foods (e.g. asparagus, bran flakes, broccoli, brussels sprouts, chick peas, dried beans, lentils, spinach, and asparagus) has even been linked to weight loss.[33] Similarly, magnesium, found naturally in avocados, bananas, beans, leafy greens, nuts, seeds, fish, whole grains, yogurt, dried fruit, and even chocolate, has been investigated for the treatment of depressive disorders. Whereas there's not enough evidence to prove magnesium supplementation works to alleviate depression, so far, the available evidence supports the use of magnesium.[34]

Many people are also convinced that omega oils are a panacea for a variety of ailments, including depression. I had a colleague who reported that he cured himself of mild depression strictly with the use of omega oils.

Indeed, research has supported the use of omega oils for the treatment of depressed mood[35] although further research is needed to support its effectiveness. In the meantime, help yourself to omega-rich foods including salmon, olive oil, flaxseed oil, eggs, evening primrose oil, avocados, nuts, and seeds. If you choose to use a supplement, consult a nutritionist so that you can be advised as to which omega oil is best and which dosage is best for you. My *Hyp2Hip Slimming* book will also provide you with insight into which foods are best for weight loss/mood lifts.

Another ingredient, a fairly expensive spice, may already be in your kitchen: saffron. This spice is used in ancient Persian traditional medicine and one that has been investigated in the treatment of depression. It has received some research support, but at this stage further research would need to identify how much is needed to treat depression effectively.[36]

As mentioned in previous chapters, amino acids seem to have a prominent place in weight management. One of them—carnitine, also known as acetyl-l-carnitine, present in meat, fish, poultry, and milk—has been trialled in the treatment of mild depression. It has been shown to be effective.[37]Another amino acid (also available as a supplement) that has shown promise as an anti-depressant as well as a weight loss agent is 5-HTP. As an anti-depressant, it has shown promise, but has not received sufficient support to be recommended.[38]

As a weight loss agent, preliminary studies have been quite impressive. A study at the University of Rome of 20 obese patients who took 900mg 5-HTP per day for 12 weeks found that 5-HTP could be effective for weight loss. Participants reported a reduction in carbohydrate intake and also reported fuller sooner. Researchers observed significant weight loss not only during the 6 week diet period, but also during the first 6 week non-diet period.[39]

Another study published in the *American Journal of Clinical Nutrition* also found 5-HTP to be effective for weight loss. Researchers put a group of obese adults on a 1,200-calorie diet and gave half of them 300 milligrams of 5-HTP to take 30 minutes before each meal. After 12 weeks, these participants lost about 7.2 pounds compared to 4 pounds in the control group.[40] Unfortunately, these and other studies on 5-HTP didn't have many participants and therefore can't be seen as conclusive evidence that 5-HTP is an effective appetite suppressant. In addition, due to a contamination problem in 1989, a batch of 5-HTP pills was linked to deaths and was consequently banned. In addition, negative interactions were reported by people who were already on anti-depressants and certain other medications, those who had liver disease, or high blood pressure.[41] Currently, 5-HTP supplements are still available on the internet.

Option 4: Herbal and homeopathic treatments

St John's Wort (Hypericum): Available in health shops and pharmacies, this plant-based treatment is sold in capsule form. It has been found to treat mild depression successfully according to a large number of placebo-controlled double-blind studies.[42] Hypericum has been found to be able to inhibit the enzymes that break down noradrenaline and serotonin just like some anti-depressants. St John's is generally well tolerated, although some people report mild side-effects such as dry mouth, dizziness, and nausea. Allergic reactions can occur in those who are generally allergic to herbs and may manifest as photo-sensitivity rashes when exposed to sunshine. I've had several of my patients report improvements after taking St John's but only those who had mild depression. From what I've seen in clinical practice, it doesn't appear to be effective in treating moderate and severe depression.

As with conventional medication, it's important to take it for long enough and in sufficient doses. Most studies demonstrating that hypericum is an effective antidepressant have used a standardised extract (6:1) of the herb. One 300mg tablet, three times daily, has been found to be the generally effective therapeutic dose, although some people will find that they only need to take one or two tablets. Also, remember the effects are not instant—according to the Black Dog Institute, St John's may take up to four weeks to exert an effect. Hypericum can interact with other medications and may not be suitable for everyone. For further information, go to the Black Dog Institute website or to www.nlm.nih.gov/medlineplus/druginfo/natural[43]

SAMe (S-Adenosyl-L-Methionine): This homeopathic treatment, available in health shops, has been used to treat depression and has been found to be effective.[44] SAMe was even trialled on 144 participants at the University of Melbourne, Department of Psychiatry. Compared to escitalopram (SSRI antidepressant), SAMe fared very well.[45] If you wish to avoid taking a conventional anti-depressant, this product may be a good option for you. I've personally used it to treat my own mild depression and felt complete relief after three weeks.

Other Herbs: A variety of other herbal remedies are available. Alternative health practitioners may recommend progesterone cream, herbs, e.g.

Vitex Agnus-Aastus and Actaea Racemosa, black cohosh, Ashwagandha, chasteberry, and vitamin and mineral supplementation. Stress management and liver detoxification (through milk thistle or Estrofactors) may also be suggested to assist the body in excreting excess estrogen. Whereas Vitex has received some research support, particularly for premenstrual dysphoric disorder, it has not received enough support to be recognised as a first line treatment.[46] If you would like to try herbal remedies, be sure to consult a trained and experienced herbalist.

Option 5: Exercise

Just when you think you will get away with not exercising ... there's another benefit of exercise that should get you even more excited about exercise. Researchers who analysed five randomised controlled trials found that exercise can relieve depression.[47] If you are struggling to get into exercise due to poor energy (in addition to lack of motivation), it may be that you need additional support to get going. In my experience of patients with depression, getting the energy to initiate exercise in the first place is difficult.

As mentioned in previous chapters, poor energy could be related to a variety of things. Whether it's low iron, low vitamin B12, stress, lack of sleep, dehydration, depression, low blood sugar, sleep apnoea, or another reason, be sure to identify and treat the cause of poor energy. You may find that getting your energy back, will make it a lot easier to exercise which will—in turn—also help relieve your depression.

Option 6: Get more sunshine

According to the phase shift hypothesis (PSH), winter depression is caused by decrease in light exposure during winter, which leads to disruption in circadian rhythms related to the sleep/wake cycle.[48] The idea of disruptions to circadian rhythms causing depression has been proven in other studies.[49] Indeed, other studies have found that mood may be correlated with daily hours of sunshine.[50] This would explain why people who do a lot of international travel (through different time zone) or people who do shift work, struggle with depression. If you live in an area like Scandinavia or the UK, which have very few hours of sunshine, you may be familiar with bright light therapy (BLT). It's a simple solution, but apparently has been found quite helpful in the treatment of SAD (seasonal depression).[51]

As you may remember from Chapter 1, vitamin D deficiency may also affect your ability to manage your weight. Because exposure to sunlight accounts for over 90 percent of the vitamin D requirement for most individuals, inadequate sunlight exposure may cause vitamin D deficiency and also restrict the antidepressant effect of light. Therefore, the link between major depression and vitamin D deficiency may be due to inadequate sunlight exposure.[52] Some researchers have even proposed that wearing sunglasses plays a role in depression.[53] Because sunshine is a good source of vitamin D and vitamin D has been linked to a depression, supplementation has also been proposed as a treatment for depression[54] Before you decide to supplement, ask your GP to test your vitamin D levels.

Other options:

A number of other things have been researched for the treatment of depression. These include (but are not limited to): avoiding alcohol, taking anti-psychotics, having ECT, Transcranial Magnetic Stimulation (TMS), ketamine, animal-assisted therapy, dance/movement therapy, acupuncture, reminiscence therapy, light therapy, massage, negative air ionisation, yoga, humour, music, singing, autogenic training, pets, melatonin, and prayer.[55] Any of these may work but don't have enough scientific evidence to support their efficacy.

Other resources for depression

Beyond Blue:
1300 224 634 or www.beyondblue.org.au
www.depression.com.au
www.reachout.com
Blue Pages depression help and resources:
www.bluepages.anu.edu.au
www.depressionnet.com.au
The Black Dog Institute:
www.blackdoginstitute.org.au

Get in the mood for weight loss:

Take the above depression questionnaires. If you believe you may have MDD or a similar disorder, do the following:

- ✓ If you are considering anti-depressants, make an appointment with a GP. You can find one by going to www.beyondblue.org.au and click on Find a Doctor
- ✓ Discuss medication options and be aware that certain anti-depressants may cause increased appetite and/ or weight gain
- ✓ If you don't want to take anti-depressants, consider St John's Wort, SAMe, or herbal supplements
- ✓ Make an appointment with a psychologist. You can find one by going to www.psychology.org.au. Read through the chapter on psychological therapy for further information.
- ✓ If your depression is mild, then try exercise
- ✓ Ensure you eat a healthy diet that is rich in vitamin D, amino acids, folate, and omega oils
- ✓ Ensure you get enough sunshine

Chapter 9: **Body Image: How to Love Your Body so It Will Love You Back**

'God grant me the serenity to change the things I can, accept the things I cannot change and the wisdom to know the difference.'
(Reinhold Niebuhr)

If you've heard of weight management experts saying, 'You have to love your body,' or, 'You can lose weight only when you love your body,' and your response is, 'But how can I love it when I hate it? I will love it only when I am slim!' then this is the chapter for you.

Body Image Defined

Body image can be defined as how you feel about your body and your appearance but also what you think about it and what actions you take as a result of this attitude about your body. These actions can be based in part by how others respond to you. How you evaluate and perceive yourself as a person has important implications for your happiness. How others perceive you can also have important consequences to you. For example, you may have difficulties finding a partner or a job because of how you feel about your appearance. Your body image can negatively affect your self-esteem. Your body image can of course also affect what you eat, whether or not or how much you exercise, what you wear, whether you feel confident to engage in new activities, etc.

Whether we like it or not, we live in a culture that evaluates someone with a lean body as having good self-control. Someone who is slim is also regarded as socially acceptable, attractive, healthy, and even competent. We are constantly inundated with images of actors, singers, and other celebrities who are—for the most part—slim! The very few exceptions are usually singled out—there is inevitably a comment about their physique. Rebel Wilson, Kate Winslet, even Cindy Crawford for being 'full-figured'.

Imagine a world in which weight and body fat was unimportant. Imagine if all that mattered was whether you were a good parent, a loving spouse, a good housekeeper, a competent employee, a kind person, an animal lover, or an adventurous person. Does it already feel better imagining this world? What if all you had to worry about in life was whether your kids were happy, whether your work was fulfilling, how much fun you could have if you were to travel to a new destination, how you could show your partner that you love him or her. *Weight Off Your Mind* will guide you to allow yourself to weigh as much or as little as you want to ... to eat what is good for you ... and to whole heartedly love yourself. First, acknowledge the facts:

How body image works

- ✓ Losing weight does not mean that you will love your body nor will it guarantee happiness
- ✓ Liposuction and bariatric surgery are unlikely to fix the psychological distress about your appearance
- ✓ Diets won't fix your poor body image either
- ✓ Recovery from Binge Eating Disorder does not guarantee improved body image
- ✓ Achieving your goal weight will not guarantee that all your other problems will be solved too

Are you surprised by some of these facts?

One more important fact about loving your body unconditionally is this:

> Accepting yourself as you are will *not* make you lose control of your eating, nor will it make you gain weight. In fact, research has proven that having a good body image may even make you lose weight and lead to improvements in your regulation of food intake.[1]

Essentially, improving your body image is a vital, not optional, component of your recovery.

Although body dysmorphic disorder has been recognised as a disorder in the Diagnostic and Statistical Manual of Disorders (DSM 5), there is no diagnosis for body image dissatisfaction. However, the following is a checklist of a list of common symptoms:

Body Image Dissatisfaction Checklist	Check if yes
Do you feel too big, fat, wide, 'frumpy', or complain about a specific part of your body? Do you refer to parts of your body in derogatory terms, e.g. 'spare tyre', 'thunder thighs', 'big, fat bum', or 'tuckshop' arms?	
Do you frequently compare yourself to others and criticise your appearance?	
Do you feel disproportionate, too tall or too short?	
Do you feel upset that your breasts are not big enough or that they are sagging or the 'wrong' shape?	
Do you feel self-conscious especially if you think people are watching you?	
Do you tend to avoid social functions because you feel too self-conscious about your body? Do you avoid the beach because you feel too embarrassed to 'expose' yourself in front of others, e.g. in swimwear?	
Do you wear clothes specifically to cover up certain body parts? Do you specifically choose certain colours (black) or certain patterns to cover up?	
Do you feel inadequate, ashamed, or embarrassed because of your body 'defects/flaws'?	
Is your distress about your body/appearance something that preoccupies your entire day on most days and is all-consuming? Have you spent a great deal of money and/or time to change your appearance?	

Body Image Dissatisfaction Checklist	Check if yes
Have you considered drastic action, e.g. liposuction or another type of surgery, in the hope to 'correct' your appearance?	
Do you tend to measure, weigh, or pinch and inspect yourself obsessively?	
Does your appearance influence your entire self-esteem?	
Have you in the past or are currently bothered by being discriminated against or teased because of your appearance? Been called 'a whale', 'fatty', 'fat chick'?	
Do you believe that most of your worries in your life are because of your appearance?	
Do you feel detached/estranged from your body?	
Do you have a chronic fear or phobia you will become fat/fatter?	
Do you feel particularly 'fat' after eating high calorie meal, premenstrually, or when you are depressed?	

Why Body Image Satisfaction is So Important

Body image satisfaction is about loving your body as it is. It's not about giving up and continuing to eat junk, binge eat or refusing to exercise. It's about accepting that despite healthy eating (including not overeating) and exercising, that you'll not achieve a perfect shape and weight but a shape and weight that's ideal for you. Body image satisfaction is also about accepting your body as it is even if it does not meet society's expectations.

Fat Acceptance and the Body Image Movement

Fat acceptance is about ending that constant battle and self-hatred just because of your shape and weight. It's about letting go of the thought of needing liposuction or anything that will change the body to conform to society's standard of what 'normal' is. It's about using the term 'fat' without thinking of it as a derogatory term. The word 'fat' is not a swearword nor an insult.

I had a friend who was considered 'painfully thin' and hated being called 'skinny' or 'thin'. Another one of my friends was very tall and hated being told she was 'Amazonian' or being made aware how tall she was—as if she didn't know it. In other words, if your hair is curly and you prefer it straight or if you are a brunette and prefer to be a blonde, it's all just about looks and something that you can change to some extent. But if you keep getting annoyed with it, then it becomes a problem.

Taryn Brumfitt, the founder of the Body Image Movement, decided that expending a great deal of effort to perfect her body was not worthwhile. She decided to cancel a tummy tuck and breast lift surgery as she came to realise that she wasn't any happier after losing 15kg and dropping from a size 10/12 to a size 6/8. She wrote two books, *Developing Daughters, Supporting Sons* and *Embrace,* which tell her story about becoming a 'body loather' to a 'body lover'. She believes it's important for her to role model having a healthy body image for her children and herself. For further information, go to www.bodyimagemovement.com.au.

Another fan of fat acceptance is Frances Lockie who writes a blog on fat acceptance. Some women go as far as preferring to be obese. They proudly belong to the 'Super-Sized Beautiful Women' (SSBW) community. They celebrate being fat; they even make money out of eating and being fat (see YouTube). Other fat acceptance supporters include Benjamin Duffy with his 'We are fat and we are legion' blog and Larson's book *Stranger Here* that outlines how weight loss surgery wasn't enough. In other words, you have the choice to simply be okay with being a size 12, 14, 16, or whatever it may be, even if society's expectation is a size 0, 6, or 8.

Is Having a Normal Body/Shape Realistic or Necessary?

Achieving your weight loss and/or eating goal may take some effort and time, especially initially. If you've lived a life of eating McDonalds because it's quick and tasty, and don't exercise because you prefer to spend your time on other things, then your weight goals is likely to backslide. It's about what you prioritise. If you prioritise your work or children or watching TV and therefore forego that hour in the gym, that's okay. But if you forego looking after yourself (and end up being a poor role model for your kids), I believe it's a problem. To me, this is all about whether you make weight loss and maintenance easy or not; surely, you have 30 minutes to take a walk (even with your kids)? If it's not an effort to eat healthily, then you can stay a size 6/8. I personally exercise no more than an hour a day and don't take longer than 30 minutes to prepare my three meals a day, so to me, weight maintenance is easy.

If you're already exercising and eating healthily and yet still can't achieve a weight that a chart or society expects you to have, then it's all about body acceptance. This is about recognising that you can change the things that are within your control and letting go of the things you can't change. In terms of whether you are in control of your weight and your eating, as you have read in previous chapters, the research on psychological therapy has provided very good evidence that it's possible to quit binge eating. It's also evident that it's possible to spot reduce with exercise and liposuction and to reduce your shape with the help of slimming machines; it's possible to improve your health with exercise and an improved diet. But is it possible to get into that ideal BMI range? Is it realistic to have a shape that society accepts as beautiful? Why was Marilyn Monroe's size 12 considered beautiful 50 years ago?

So, we know that we can do something to change the shape of our bodies. There's also a large body of scientific evidence that supports the notion that our environment influences what and how much we eat. However, there's also evidence that our genes affect appetite, satiety, metabolism, food cravings, body-fat distribution, and the tendency to use food as a coping tool. A study (of more than 900 people) that was published in the journal *Science* found that those who have two copies of a specific gene 'Insig-2' were 22 percent more likely to have a BMI over 30.[2]

Twin studies have found that genetic factors explain 50-90 percent of the difference in our weight. Family studies (parent, child, or sibling) range from 20 to 80 percent. Data from adoption studies are consistent with genetic factors accounting for 20 to 60 percent of the variation in BMI.[3] If you are interested in discovering if genes play a role in your inability to lose weight, read an interesting report in Harvard Health at www.health.harvard.edu/WL.

Dr Bouchard of the Pennington Biomedical Research Centre at Louisiana State University said there are over 100 genes responsible for obesity. Recent research has found that people who inherit FTO gene—responsible for metabolism—are 60 percent more likely to be obese if they have two copies of the gene. Those with just 1 copy are overweight.[4]

But just in case you're thinking your genes have cursed you for life, remember that even alcoholics, who are known to have a gene specific to their illness, can recover from alcoholism. In other words, genetics helps determine your natural weight range, but you have some control over where you fall within that range.[5] A study on 144 participants has concluded that those people who were overweight in childhood are particularly resistant to treatment that targets weight.[6] Thus, recognising that your genes may be going against you in terms of achieving an 'ideal' body weight, bear in mind that you are not giving up by accepting your body as it is. Do the following exercises to improve your body image.

8 Steps To Supersize Your Body Confidence

Step 1: Correct your body image, not your appearance

Has stressing about your appearance helped you? If you still believe that just correcting those flaws through surgery will make you feel better about yourself, think again: according to research at University of Pittsburgh Weight Management Center, body contouring post bariatric surgery to correct loose skin improved body image but produced dis-satisfaction with other parts of the body![7]

Rather than focusing on 'correcting' your appearance, focus instead on correcting your body image, which can in fact, have a positive effect on your eating. In fact,

> Researchers in Portugal of 239 overweight women found that treatment that addresses body image dissatisfaction has beneficial effects on eating behaviour. They concluded that the best outcomes would come from therapy that helps a person reduce the importance of their body/weight in their lives.[8]

Thus, you're better off with psychological therapy than surgery.

Step 2: Do desensitisation exercises

One of the best ways to overcome body dissatisfaction is to do exactly those things that you are avoiding. Well known body image treatment researchers recommend that people with body image concerns should learn to accept (not necessarily like) their current body shape and engage in activities they have avoided because of their embarrassment about their body.[9] For example, if you are currently avoiding looking into the mirror: do it now! If you're currently avoiding undressing in front of your partner, do just that! How about having a shower in a public shower, going to the beach in a bikini, or even accepting a compliment? If you're thinking you could never do this: try it—see if it works. What's the worst that could happen? Would you experience shame, embarrassment, and anxiety? Probably. However, with repeated attempts, you will find that this anxiety will ease.

One of my patients told me that she feared if she got undressed in front of her partner that he would reject her or not be 'turned on'. Asked how she would feel about being with a man who rejected her for her looks, she stated: 'I would be devastated losing him,' but upon further reflection said, 'Why would I want to be with someone who doesn't love me unconditionally?' I understand doing something you've avoided for fear of shame, embarrassment or anxiety is not easy. If you're struggling to implement these avoided behaviours, psychological therapy is indicated.

Step 3: Accept that you're not perfect and may be normal after all

Body image is a subjective judgment and yet the media continues to suggest that if you're not skinny, you're not normal and in fact, unacceptable. In case you don't already know: photoshopping of people in magazines is commonplace. In fact, magazine editors are famous for insisting that images be photoshopped. To us, it appears that all women have big breasts, a tiny waist, cellulite-free, stretch-mark free long legs, a smooth blemish-free wrinkle-free face, and a perfectly proportioned body. If you don't look like that, you need to buy a pill, a cream, certain make up, have surgery, spend thousands on a diet program, etc.

Sadly, photoshopping is almost a given. Even my photographer, who took shots of me for my professional website, asked me if I preferred the altered photo he sent—the one he altered using a program called 'Portrait Professional' that automatically corrects flaws. I refused. So, I have a few lines on my face and I am not a size 0. I don't care.

Research has confirmed that watching images of idealised skinny people on TV and in magazines or any sort of media is associated with eating disorders, poor self-esteem, negative emotions, and of course, body dissatisfaction.[10]

I remember a few years ago that Tanya Plibersek, a former minister of health, had made recommendations to the media to avoid the perpetuation of media-induced eating disorders but was unable to make it mandatory. You can learn more about the movement to stop photoshopping in media images by going to websites 'Keep it Real' and 'Miss Representation'.

So far, the Keep It Real campaign is targeting the editors of numerous magazines including *Cosmopolitan, Lucky, Teen Vogue,* and *Marie Claire*. People are urged to join a Facebook event page that says: 'I'm taking the Keep It Real Challenge. It's time for the media to drop Photoshop and show real beauty.' Alternatively, you can also do other things, e.g. start a petition on Change.org to insist that modelling agencies and magazine editors stop using skinny models and take needed action to stop the perpetuation of the thin ideal.

In the meantime, avoid all magazines that have thin models. If you have any magazines in your house with those thin ideals in them, throw them out. Take out a subscription to a magazines that stimulate your mind and make you happy and never read those other magazines in any waiting room!

Step 4: Focus on health, not appearance

You know by now that being skinny will not necessarily make you happy or happier. But did you know that there's also some controversy as to whether losing weight will actually make you healthier? We are constantly bombarded with messages in the media that being obese and even overweight is unhealthy. The medical profession has forwarded several pieces of evidence linking all sorts of diseases with excess fat, yet others have proposed that better health is not necessarily achieved by reduced weight.[11]

US-based cardiologist Dr Lavi based at John Ochsner Heart and Vascular Institute, author of the book *The Obesity Paradox: when thinner means sicker and heavier means healthier,* says that fitness is more important than thinness. He has found evidence that compared to those who have heart disease, the overweight, and moderately obese are better off, citing a 30-50 percent lower mortality rates than lean people who have these diseases. The idea that being fit is (even when overweight or obese) is healthier than being slim was found by other researchers too.[11]

In addition, according to researchers at York University in Toronto and in an article published in *Obesity Reviews*, there is increasing evidence that those with heart disease or diabetes, weight cyclers, metabolically healthy obese adults, youth, older adults, or 'fit and fat' individuals are not negatively affected by their increased fat; neither would they benefit from weight loss.[12]

Regardless of whether or not you have a genetic predisposition toward being obese or overweight, research with 20,000 people has confirmed that you can reduce your genetic propensity for obesity by about 40 percent by being physically active.[13] What researchers have found is that even if you don't lose weight, the beneficial effects of exercise on cardiometabolic risk factors keeps you healthy.

This is because even one acute bout of exercise can significantly reduce insulin sensitivity, cholesterol, blood pressure, blood glucose, and triglycerides.[14] What this means for you is if you're happy with your weight (even it's it's not a 'normal' weight), you don't have to stress about it. However, do continue to eat healthy foods and exercise.

Step 5: Stop criticising, comparing and scrutinising your body

I've had a few patients come into therapy who were unhappy with their appearance despite having quit binge eating. Some of them have expressed fear that having therapy to be content with their bodies will make them put on weight. Is this your fear? If so, rest assured: research has proven this is not the case.[15]

> Improving your body image will not make you gain weight

Consider taking on a fresh perspective by acknowledging that you are more than your appearance. Identify all the positive qualities you have. Detach your self-esteem from your weight. Instead of comparing your body with another person's, look at other qualities you like about another person.

Step 6: Stop attributing all your problems to your weight/shape

If you've been in the habit of blaming everything bad about life on your weight, open your eyes and see now that your problems could be attributed to other things. Identify what else may be the problem. Think about how you would spend your day if you weren't worrying about dieting, your weight, and shape.

Step 7: Learn to cope with criticism and judgment from others

First impressions are important and are made within seconds of meeting you and are usually made from your appearance. People may judge you negatively because of your shape/weight or they may do so because of your personality or other features. However, you also know that the friends you have at the moment love you and may not have had a bad initial impression of you. Essentially, your appearance is important for initial impressions to unacquainted people only.

Whereas it would be very difficult to change everyone's perception of 'fat' people, you can change the way you cope with negative remarks or discrimination by others. Or, have you recognised that sometimes the way people treat you is not solely because of your weight or that you are not the only person being targeted? If you're unable to conform to the conventional beauty ideal, your option is to learn to cope with criticism and judgment from others. This may not be easy, so if you are struggling with this particular problem, I would recommend attending psychological therapy.

In the USA, there is more activity to counteract weight discrimination. If you're interested in this campaign, have a look at the following:

- The National Association to Advance Fat Acceptance www.NAAFA.org
- The Association for the Health Enrichment of Large People (AHELP)
- The Network for Size Esteem www.eskimo.com/~largesse
- www.largelypositive.com

- www.healthweightnetwork.com
- www.radiancemagazine.com

Step 8: Find happiness regardless of your shape and weight

Did you know that achieving your desired/ideal goal weight or shape will not make you happier? Indeed, according to a study at the University College of London of almost 2,000 overweight and obese adults, those who lost at least 5 percent of their body weight were healthier but not necessarily happy.[16] Just as I have had addicts in my office believing all their problems will be resolved once they are sober, I've had obese binge eaters thinking that all will be well once their weight and fat is in order. Apparently, winning the lotto too is not associated with greater happiness in the long run either.[17]

As I have emphasised throughout this book, dieting alone, without addressing other problems associated with your weight problem, is unlikely to lead to long term weight management. Neither will it make you suddenly be happy with your body. In fact, as I pointed out earlier, dieting and its inevitable failure, is likely to make you less happy—confirmed many times in research.[18]

Does constantly worrying about your health not cause disease? If achieving your ideal weight and shape would lead to unbridled happiness, I would definitely recommend losing weight and doing whatever it takes. I personally am happier that I've lost the weight I wanted to and feel that happiness every time I get undressed or dressed, walk around in public. I feel happy and empowered when I eat rather than overeat or binge eat. It's a goal I've achieved, not something that was given to me. That, to me, is the reason I'm happy about conquering the weight and eating problem. To others perhaps, I could still lose more weight, get rid of the stretch marks or the cellulite but it's not something that would make me happy/happier. If you're aware that achieving your ideal body won't necessarily make you happier, but you still want to achieve it, go for it. But if you recognise that you may be thin/thinner but not happier, also know that you can still benefit from improving your body image.

Many books on happiness will explain how to become happy. Although actively pursuing a goal can improve your happiness, it's also important to remember that achieving your weight goal will not eliminate all other things you may be unhappy about. If you would like to be happier, I recommend reading any books on happiness, e.g. *The How of Happiness* by Sonja Lyubomirsky. If you would like further information about body image therapy:

- www.healthnotdiets.com
- *The Non-Diet Approach Guidebook* (Adams and Willer)
- *The Body Image Workbook: an 8 step program for Learning to like your Looks* (Cash)

Chapter 10: **How to Overcome Food Addiction, Binge Eating, and Emotional Eating**

'Food is like sex: when you abstain even the worst food begins to look good.'
(Beth McCollister)

A study reported in *Obesity Review* (2005) found that people who maintain their weight after weight loss tend not to binge eat or overeat.[1] Research from the National Weight Control Registry also found that maintainers don't binge eat.[2] In other words, the mentality of 'being good' for a few days and then 'blowing out' is not present. Maintainers have a consistent eating pattern across weekdays and weekends. Binge eating can be part of a psychological disorder, Binge Eating Disorder. Fortunately, this chapter will provide you with the tools to overcome this problem.

A study has shown that those with Binge Eating Disorder attained only 55 percent of the weight loss that non-binge eaters attained.[3]

The Drug/Food Addiction Parallel

If you are like most people with a weight problem, eating 'normally' is hard to do. Although most eating disorder researchers will disagree with the term 'addiction' when it comes to food, I can clearly see the similarities between food and drug addiction. When I worked in a drug rehabilitation centre, I spoke to an alcoholic who asked me, 'How is it that someone can walk into a bar, drink half the one beer he ordered, and walk out?' That—to me—was the equivalent of a binge eater saying, 'How is it that someone can buy a family block of chocolate, eat two pieces, and put the rest away?'

Life as a Food Addict—can you relate to some of these?

- ✓ I eat because I cannot stop—the urge takes hold of me just like a junkie who craves another fix
- ✓ I eat in one sitting what 'normal' people may not even eat in one day
- ✓ I eat more only because it tastes good or to treat myself
- ✓ I eat even though I have just eaten or just because someone has offered it
- ✓ I eat because there is an urge that takes hold of me like a tornado
- ✓ I eat despite the guilt that engulfs me afterwards
- ✓ I eat because food is my best friend
- ✓ I eat junk food not because I don't know better but because I just cannot see the appeal of a salad
- ✓ I eat because I feel sad or upset or because I can't cope with the real problems
- ✓ I will eat to the point of nausea or feeling uncomfortably full

- ✓ I eat strange mixtures of things (e.g. dates with cream) or thicken things to make it more filling
- ✓ When I run out of food, I will eat anything in the pantry, even if it's chewable vitamins or dog or cat food
- ✓ I sometimes eat food that is still frozen/raw/too hot/with wrapping, because I can't wait for it to get ready
- ✓ I sometimes pretend to buy a cake 'for guests', then go home and eat it all by myself
- ✓ I will drive to the petrol station or convenience store just to get binge food even late at night
- ✓ When I go grocery shopping I can't wait to go home to eat it, so I eat it while driving
- ✓ I'm so glad nobody sees me when I binge, because of the amount I eat but also because of the way I just shovel it in there (really bad table manners)
- ✓ I'm sometimes so desperate to eat that I will eat something even if it's food scraps, been in the garbage bin, or on a dirty floor
- ✓ I eat just because

Does that sound like you? Research has identified that if you are male, you are more likely to be 'addicted' to steaks and roasts, hamburgers, french fries, pizza, and ice cream, whereas if you are a female, you're more likely to be 'addicted' to bread, cake, cookies, ice cream, chocolate, pies, and other desserts. Addictions to these foods that raise endorphin levels are common, as eating these foods enhances the body's natural pleasure providers.[4]

If you were to look at the way you behave around food the same way a drug addict behaves around drugs, can may be able to relate to this:

Drug/alcohol addiction criteria[5]	**Food addiction parallel**
Tolerance: need for more of a substance to achieve the same effect or a diminished effect when using the same amount of the substance over time, e.g. needing 10 beers to get drunk rather than only 4 beers to get drunk	Not feeling full/satisfied with a regular portion, needing to eat oversized portions
Withdrawal: shaking, sweating, anxiety when no alcohol is available	Feeling deprived, irritable, or distressed when (the binge) food is not available
Using more than intended or for longer than intended	Eating more than intended
Repeated unsuccessful attempts to reduce or persistent desire to do so	Repeated unsuccessful attempts to eat less or diet or persistent desire to do so
Substantial amount of time spent obtaining, using, or recovering from use	Eating fast in an attempt to feel full and feeling nauseous, bloated following meals; grazing all day
Drug use is prioritised over recreational, work, or family activities	Eating is done while watching TV or at other times that eating should not occur; eating venues and events are sought out in favour of sports; eating occurs in secret
Use continued despite physical or psychological consequences	Overeating/bingeing occurs despite diabetes, gallstones, high cholesterol, hyper-tension (or other physical diseases), poor body image, and poor self-esteem

As early as the 1950s, certain kinds of overeating patterns were being compared to addictions.[6] In a study on obesity conducted by a psycho-analytically-oriented psychiatrist in 1959, eight of eighteen patients were categorised as displaying 'an intense kind of craving for food which is insatiable' ... The analogy to alcohol and other addictions is appropriate both in terms of the behaviour and the personality structure of these patients'.[6]

Understanding Food Addiction Fact #1: Your Brain Reacts Abnormally To Food

Abnormal eating patterns in humans appear to be associated with specific disturbances in brain neuro-chemical function, according to an article in the *Psychiatry Research.*[7] Translated: your brain is wired differently! If you've ever wondered why you have sweet cravings, you may be relieved to know that you're not 'just a sweet tooth'. Researchers have found sweet cravings may be due to the fact that overweight and obese people are more sensitive to immediate rewards and thus experience food as more pleasurable and rewarding than 'normal' weight people.[8]

On the other hand, other researchers have found that overeating and bingeing may be a person's response to gain pleasure from eating when it has been blunted.[9] Similarly, research with Positron Emission Tomography (PET) have shown that obese people have significantly fewer pleasure receptors compared with normal weight people.[10] Low levels of pleasure receptors are found not only in people with a high BMI but also in chronic drug and alcohol use users.[11]

Researchers have actually coined the term 'reward deficiency syndrome' to describe this phenomenon (of low numbers pleasure receptors) and say it leads people to engage compulsively in rewarding behaviours such as drug use and eating.[12] Not only sweet foods, but very tasty calorie rich foods stimulates the feel good brain chemical dopamine leading to feelings of pleasure.[13]

The fact that opioid antagonist medications meant for drug addicts work for binge eaters also indicates that a similar process is involved. For example, Naloxone, used for the treatment of drug addiction, has been found to be useful for binge eaters. More specifically, sensory preferences for sugar/fat mixtures and the consumption of sweets are reduced by infusions of naloxone.[14]

If there is indeed such a thing as food addiction, what this means for you in terms of recovery from it, based on the model of addiction, is total abstinence. Whereas obviously you can't abstain from food totally, food addicts are advised to avoid the food they feel addicted to, e.g. from sugar, wheat, etc. Before you go into panic, remember that this abstinence model is just one particular approach. Just as there is a moderation model for alcoholics, so too is there a moderation model for food addicts. I personally have found patients do well with complete abstinence from sugar and/or wheat, for example, but I've also had patients who have done well with moderating their favourite food. There's a whole chapter on how to enjoy your favourite food. The *Hyp2Hip Slimming* book also has a section that enlightens you about the concept of sugar not being the enemy. Remember: *Weight Off Your Mind* is about changing the way you think about food, eating, and your body. It's not about banning your favourite food. It's about letting you be emotionless about food.

Understanding Food Addiction Fact #2: Food Scientists and Manufacturers Engulf You in an Obesogenic Space

A drug/alcohol counsellor will always advise an alcoholic in recovery to stay away from a bar or other environment in which alcohol is not around. Is it that easy for us binge eaters? Can you walk around the street without seeing food at least advertised? Can you walk into a grocery store without seeing your 'drug'—whether it's chocolate, bread, or any food at all? No, because essentially we are surrounded by food or food messages very frequently—an 'obesogenic' environment.

A symposium at Purdue University Ingestive Behavior Research Center presented the research about the difference between 'thrifty' and 'high fat phenotype' people. They found that some people exposed to an obesogenic environment remain lean. Others respond to the same environment quite differently: they don't feel satiated after eating fatty meals, have a preference for high-fat foods (even when satiated), eat for pleasure (especially tasty foods), and have a tendency to eat without inhibitions.[15]

In other words, as a food addict, it's incredibly difficult to avoid foods in an 'obesogenic' environment in which we are exposed to food all the time: on TV we are exposed to food adverts—mostly junk food. We are encouraged to eat everywhere we go: in cinemas we are offered giant sized popcorn and 'jumbo' sized soft drinks; we walk around and see food advertised; we drive on the street and see food advertised; at buffet style restaurants, we are encouraged to 'eat all you can'.

Marketers have made it an art form to make us buy and eat foods we wouldn't normally have. Why, for example, are the foods highest in sugar or fat placed at eye-level in supermarkets? Why do supermarkets place chocolates at the register when you are standing right in front of them, staring at them, with that waiting time a perfect opportunity to add them to your trolley? Why do food manufacturers get away with labelling a product 'reduced fat' fooling us into thinking it is low fat when in fact in may only be 25 percent less fat than the original product? How is it they can label foods with monosodium glutamate making us think it doesn't contain salt?

But food scientists too have mastered the science of making food more palatable so that we eat more and buy more because we enjoy it more. When my father had a herb and spice manufacturing company, his food scientist told me that she was taught many ways to increase pleasure from foods, e.g. by contrasting different textures, e.g. crunchy with soft; making foods 'melt' in your mouth; mixing different flavours, e.g. salt and sugar, sweet and sour; and adding ingredients like fat to enhance the flavour. All those tricks make foods irresistible.

Food scientist Steven Witherly makes a very interesting observation about this in his report 'Why Humans Like Junk Food'. Michael Moss, too, in his book *Salt, Sugar, Fat* exposes how the food industry has us hooked on certain foods all for their profit. So, if you think you choose foods only because of what they look like, whether they are available, how affordable you think they are, and whether or not you like the quality and brand, think again. You have been deceived.

Understanding Food Addiction Fact #3: You May Have a Disorder

If someone were to tell a diabetic person to 'just stop having insulin problems, pull yourself together!' would you think that's not the right response? But that is what binge eaters are told, 'just eat less and exercise more!' We are treated like freaks. But yes, Binge Eating Disorder is an actual disorder, just like diabetes.

Whereas a huge amount of research supports the theory of 'food addiction', most eating disorder experts talk in terms of Binge Eating Disorder (BED) and classify it as a mental health disorder. BED has been a formal diagnosis in the 'Diagnostic and Statistical Manual of Mental Health Disorder' (DSM-5) only since the last edition was published in 2013. In previous editions, Binge Eating Disorder was only known as an 'eating disorder not otherwise specified'.

Binge Eating Disorder Checklist (BED)	Check if yes
1. Do you binge eat? i.e. eat large amount of food in a short amount of time, e.g. eat a whole packet of chips or a whole carton of biscuits	
2. Do you have a sense of lack of control over your food intake?	
Continue to question 3 only if both 1 and 2 occur	
3. Do you eat quickly?	
4. Do you eat until you are uncomfortably full?	

Binge Eating Disorder Checklist (BED)	Check if yes
5. Do you eat even when not hungry? e.g. when you are bored, anxious, just because it is there?	
6. Do you eat alone due to being embarrassed about your eating?	
7. Do you feel disgusted, embarrassed, or depressed about your eating?	
If you have checked at least 3 of questions 3-7, continue to question 8.	
8. Do you feel great distress about your eating?	
If yes, continue to question 9.	
9. Have you been binge eating at least once weekly the past 3 months?	
If yes, continue to question 10.	
10. Do you tend to avoid compensating for your bingeing by taking laxatives, vomiting, or excessive exercise?	
If yes, you may have Binge Eating Disorder.	
Severity: mild (1-3 binges per week), moderate (4-7 binges per week), severe (8-13 binges per week), extreme (14+ binges per week).	
Note: the difference between bingeing and overeating is that overeating simply involves eating a large amount whereas bingeing means eating a large amount but also having a sense of losing control over eating.	

**This questionnaire was based on the DSM-5 criteria for Binge Eating Disorder[16] but should not be used to self-diagnose. It should be used as a guide only. Only a qualified mental health practitioner (psychologist, psychiatrist) can diagnose BED.*

Another feature of Binge Eating Disorder (BED) is 'the overvaluation of weight or shape', which means you tend to think your weight and shape is more important than other things. Some people with BED also have 'general psychological distress' or other mental health symptoms, e.g. depression, anxiety. Some also find interactions with others difficult.[17]

Strangely lacking in the BED diagnostic criteria is the concept of poor body image. However, researchers have identified that some people with BED engage in a great deal of body checking and avoidance.[18] In my clinical experience with people with BED, most of them have a body hatred that affects all areas of their lives: their sex life in particular, but even their daily lives involves feeling uncomfortable buying clothes and looking in the mirror.

BED is often associated with severe illnesses and mortality due to its link to obesity. Whereas not all people with BED are obese or even overweight, it most often leads to obesity. More than 65 percent of BED patients are obese but not all obese people have BED—in fact, BED occurs in about 10 percent of obese people.[19]

The causes of BED have been investigated in many studies. Fairburn, a well-known eating disorder expert, did a study of 52 women with BED and 104 without an eating disorder and 102 with other psychological disorders. He identified that people are more at risk of developing BED if they have:

- Negative childhood experiences
- Parental depression
- Vulnerability to obesity
- Repeated exposure to negative comments about shape, weight, and eating[20]

The above findings are similar to a report published in the *Obesity Reviews* journal, which stated that children are at particular risk of BED when they grow up in a disharmonious family environment, where they are exposed to parental frustrations (e.g. arguments about money or the relationship), do not have support, have negative belief systems, and unmet emotional needs.[21] The report also explains how these factors, combined with poor resilience (and poor coping skills), lead to poor self-esteem, a sense of powerlessness, depression, anxiety, and decreased stress tolerance. Eating is then adopted as a coping tool.

Researchers have also identified that for many emotional eaters, mealtimes were turbulent—described as control battles between parent and child.[22] Food consequently became associated with control. Eating subsequently became a way to gain control over other aspects of life. Eating also became a way to numb the pain associated with child abuse or to substitute for human needs for relationship and belonging. Can you relate to this?

Understanding Food Addiction Fact #4: You Cope by Eating

Do you use the term 'emotional eating' or 'comfort eating' when you mean that you are eating not because you are truly hungry? Do you eat for emotional reasons? e.g. grieving, frustration, boredom, depression, loneliness, guilt (tension and regret for having done something wrong), shame (feeling like a bad person for having done something wrong). Are these feelings brought on by stressors?—perhaps about being overweight and feeling desperate about problematic eating, but also by stressors including family problems, pain and health issues, financial problems, relationship problems, poor self-esteem, general stress, conflict, inability to cope with demands at home or work, quitting smoking, trauma related to natural disasters, sexual or physical abuse, or conflict and lack of pleasure. Some researchers have also proposed that people may misattribute perceived stress to eating in order to distract from the original source of distress.[23] In other words, there's a major stressor going on in your life, but you believe your stress is related to your eating.

One of my patients who came to me for weight management, said, 'I don't really engage in emotional eating'. She explained that she just eats when she feels hungry. She said she used to feel hungry 'all the time' even shortly after eating a meal but in the past few years has gotten a bit better, feeling hungry mostly in the evening after dinner and had cravings for chocolate premenstrually. Asked what she was eating, she explained, 'One block of chocolate, polished off in 5 minutes, or if there's no chocolate, a pantry or fridge raid of whatever was there: cereal, rice or bread.'

We explored her idea that this was *not* emotional eating. She argued that she does not eat because she feels bored, sad, lonely, or otherwise emotional. She eats because she is 'really hungry'. She eventually realised that even though she did not identify a specific emotion other than *hunger*, it was a hunger that was out of the ordinary for her caloric and nutritional requirements. She agreed that her hunger was extreme and abnormal, not actual hunger. She agreed this was, in fact, 'emotional' hunger. I had another patient who said she, 'Subconsciously ate to get fat because the last time I lost weight, I got lots of attention from men—which was problematic as my husband got really jealous and verbally abused me.' She ate for protection, she said. Again, eating for emotional reasons, not for nutritional or caloric needs.

Alcoholics Anonymous has a good acronym to halt alcoholics from thinking they need an alcoholic drink: HALT. First ask: are you **H**ungry, **A**ngry, **L**onely or **T**ired? If so, you can do something about that, e.g. eat when you hungry; talk and resolve the things you are angry about; phone a friend if you are lonely; and make sure you get enough sleep. All these things alert the person to the fact it's not in fact a craving for alcohol—it's a feeling and you can do something other than drink to ease it. The way this translates to binge eating is to ask yourself: am I really hungry or am I feeling angry, tired, lonely ... thirsty, sad, irritated? If so, do something about it (except eat).

Are you eating because you're hungry or eating to change how you feel?

A review of the literature published in the *International Journal of Eating Disorders* and a report in *Eating Behaviours* have confirmed that overweight people have higher rates of emotional eating when they're feeling an uncomfortable emotion compared to healthy-weight individuals.[24] According to a study in *Appetite*, emotional eaters tend to expect that food will make them feel better and therefore keep eating because just eating 'one cookie' has not delivered the desired result. [25]

In psychology, we use the term 'cognitive appraisal' to describe how we interpret things. For example, if you usually overeat in response to an uncomfortable feeling such as anger or sadness, you may have then appraise/label food as being positive because food soothed you. The more often you use food as a coping tool, the less likely you are to activate the part of your brain that has alternative coping mechanisms. Although you may have an alternative coping mechanism, it remains dormant and are thus unable to use it. It's the same as the 'use it or lose it' principle. This puts you at high risk for relapse when you encounter stress.[26] But researchers have also found that some emotional eaters also eat in response to being in a happy mood.[27] This, of course, is also a problem as you will then be triggered to eat whether you feel happy or sad.

Generally, emotional eating is understood to be a complex behaviour associated with:

- Poor self-esteem[28]
- Poor coping strategies[29]
- Low satisfaction with basic needs[30].
- Desire to reduce anxiety[31]

Researchers have also found that emotional eaters are more sensitive to rewards (i.e. food) when they are feeling an uncomfortable emotion. Unfortunately, despite binging, all that food doesn't necessarily do the job of alleviating the negative feelings.[32] This is probably the reason you feel unsatisfied even though you have eaten in attempt to escape from negative feelings. In addition, eating 'forbidden' food may also cause guilt,[33] especially if you're a woman,[34] making it even more of a vicious cycle.

Earlier researchers theorised that obese people had 'faulty hunger awareness' and had incorrectly learned the signals for hunger, thus feeling the same if they were hungry or uncomfortable emotionally, causing them to eat in both situations.[35] It is now common knowledge that some people eat due to difficulty differentiating between hunger cues and emotional arousal. Do you struggle with this?

A diet or bariatric surgery is not the cure for emotional eating ... and neither is a biscuit, or twenty!

2 Steps to Overcome Problem Eating

Step 1: Do not blame yourself

As you have read above: your experiences as a child as well as your biology has made your brain respond differently to food compared to a normal weight person. Food scientists have hooked you in with their 'black magic' food science and the food industry has manipulated you, placing you in an obesogenic environment in which you are always exposed to tasty, fattening food. You are not alone: you have a disorder that is prevalent in a least four percent of the population.[36] The good news is that BED is treatable. As mentioned in the chapter on psychological therapy and alternative therapy, there are many options. You're not trapped. You're not the puppet. Never ever blame yourself. Start treatment to get yourself out of the spinning webs of the food industry.

Step 2: Learn coping skills and rewire your brain to alleviate problem eating

You may have now digested the fact that improving coping skills can greatly reduce the need to engage in emotional eating,[37] especially if you eat to cope with life stressors. The chapter on psychological therapy may be useful to guide you in the right direction with this. It is time now to climb Mount Recovery and view life from the top!

My recommendation is that you attend psychological therapy if you are chronically binge eating. If you would like further information about eating disorders and food addiction, go to:

- The Food Addiction Institute, which has a list of 2,734 citations that includes peer reviewed scientific journals about chemical dependency on food and the biochemical effects of sugar, fat, and caffeine interacting with dopamine and serotonin receptors. It also includes studies of other biochemical mechanisms including leptin deficiency curtailing satiation, glycemic and insulin malfunctions, and allergies to wheat and other foods. Over 100 citations are texts about obesity, eating disorders, or addiction. It also includes a list of texts of self-help treatments of food addiction and cookbooks eliminating addictive foods. The rest are clinical studies including case studies of recovered food addicts, research on the effectiveness of food-related twelve step programs, quantitative outcome research on food addiction treatment programs, and qualitative research on food addiction denial.
- The Eating Disorders Association Qld: www.eda.org.au
- Overcoming Overeating: www.overcomingover-eating.com
- Overeaters Anonymous: www.oa.org/index.htm
- Various eating disorder websites:
    - www.ceed.org.au
    - www.cci.health.wa.gov.au
    - www.eatingdisorders.org.au

- www.somethingfishy.org
- www.thebutterflyfoundation.org.au
- www.edauk.com
- www.isis.org.au
- www.recoveryispossible.com.au
- www.smart-eating.com
- www.mentorconnect-ed.org
- http://au.reachout.com/find/articles/binge-eating-disorder
- www.stopcompulsiveeating.com/faq.php
- www.addictionrecoveryguide.org
- www.edreferral.com
- www.treatyourselfwell.com.au

- The Skinny of Obesity by Dr Lustig (TV program)
- Books:
  - *Overcoming Binge Eating* (Fairburn)
  - *The Binge Eating and Compulsive Overeating Workbook* (Ross)
  - *Feeding The Hungry Heart: The experience of compulsive eating* (Geneen)
  - *When Women Stop Hating Their Bodies* (Munter & Hirschmann)
  - *The Addicted Brain & How to Break Free* (Kessler)
  - *Food Triggers* (Epstein)
- For information on how to read and understand food labels, go to www.foodstandards.gov.au

Chapter 11: **Forbidden Fruit—How to Eat Your Favourite Food**

'Food imaginatively and lovingly prepared, and eaten in good company, warms the being.'
(Marjorie Kinnan Rawlings)

If you have Binge Eating Disorder and/or struggle with your weight, food, and eating, you are likely to be familiar with ambivalent feelings around food. On the one hand, you feel pleasure and enjoyment; on the other, worry and guilt. Guilt has the potential to motivate behaviour change, but may also lead to feelings of helplessness and loss of control. For example, if you feel guilty about not helping a friend in need, it is likely to motivate you to ask a friend whether he or she needs your assistance. However:

> If you feel guilty about eating a certain food, it can lead to bingeing.

Does that sound like you? This chapter will provide you with the insight that you need to be in control of your favourite food and provide you with guidelines on how to eat your favourite food without guilt and loss of control. *Weight Off Your Mind* is about letting you eat anything you want rather than restricting you to a certain way of eating. It's about establishing or re-establishing a healthy relationship with food rather than making you evaluate a certain food as 'good' or 'bad' and going on the diet round-about again and again.

The best way to lose weight is not to find the best diet; it's to release worry, concern and guilt about food.

6 Joyous Paths to Have Your Cake and Eat It

Joyous path to slimness step 1: Stop eating with guilt

Your joyous path to slimness will involve learning that you can eat alone, at restaurants, parties, with family, with friends ... anywhere, anyhow but never with guilt. Research published in *Appetite* confirmed that your weight loss is unlikely to be successful if you associate guilt with eating.[1] This was confirmed by a particular study in which participants were asked whether they felt 'guilt' or 'celebration' with a forbidden food item (e.g. chocolate cake). They examined if their attitude was related to perceived behavioural control, intentions to eat healthily, and whether they were able to lose weight over an 18 month period (and short term weight-loss in a subsample of participants with a weight-loss goal). Participants associating chocolate cake with guilt did not report more positive attitudes or stronger intentions to eat healthy than those associating chocolate cake with celebration. Instead, they reported lower levels of perceived behavioural control over eating and were less successful at maintaining their weight over an 18-month period. Weight-loss goal participants who associated chocolate cake with guilt were less successful at losing weight over a 3-month period compared to those associating chocolate cake with celebration.

This finding is similar to the 'milkshake study' that confirms that it's our perception rather than an actual substance that affects us, i.e., if people perceive a food to be 'indulgent', they experience it as more satisfying compared to a food they perceive as 'sensible', even it has the same calorie content. The perception of it even influences the way hunger hormones respond! It's from this that we know that there is no such thing as 'evil' food. It's only your perception. Thus, here is your instruction on how to eat your favourite food—EAT IT! But eat it only without guilt.

> The more guilty you feel about eating chocolate, the more likely you are to feel out of control of your eating behaviour and the less likely you are to achieve weight maintenance.

Joyous path to slimness step 2: Stop the 'what-the-hell effect'/all or nothing thinking and behaviour

Not only does dietary restriction increase desire for forbidden foods in the form of craving, it also tends to induce guilt, anxiety, and depression. Research shows us a psychological phenomenon happens when a person believes he or she has eaten a forbidden, binge, or 'bad' food. He or she engages in 'disinhibited eating' in which all-or-nothing thinking occurs, leading to a total binge.[2] Typically it sounds like: 'I've had a piece of chocolate cake, I've blown it. I may as well have the whole cake then.' Can you relate to this?

Try NOT to have it and you will be drawn to it all the more.

This is a psychological principle called 'paradoxical intention'. I had a patient who came to me weighing 116kg. She told me, 'I try not to have chocolate, ice cream, or biscuits.' She told me of what her typical diet consisted. While I believed a dietitian may have tweaked her diet a bit to include more vegetables and less protein, I could not see how she could have been that overweight. In the first session I asked her what her favourite foods were. She replied, 'Ice cream, chocolate, biscuits ... and some fruit.' I told her to have exactly that. She returned the following week and said, 'When I left the session last week, I felt I was in a haze of bliss. I sat down on a park bench and thought, 'This isn't me.' She told me how she had told her husband that I had prescribed her to eat whatever she wanted and ordered him to not nag her about eating chocolates, biscuits, and ice cream. She proceeded to eat biscuits, ice cream, and chocolate and in one instance walked out of the grocery store thinking, *I didn't even buy chocolate! I don't even want chocolate*. Asked what her weight was, she said, 'It's the same. Before I would've put on a kg if I'd eaten like this.' All this without hypnosis! Just by giving her permission to eat *like a slim person!*

As long as you have 'forbidden' foods on your list, food is in control of you, food is the enemy, and you are constantly at war with it. *Weight Off Your Mind* is about letting you be the master. Dog behaviourists, for example, say that a dog that is not well behaved is because the dog owner has not trained the dog. Once the owner is trained how to manage the dog, the dog will be well behaved. Your mind functions in the same way: when you are trained how to behave around food, you will be 'well behaved' around food. If you find yourself having a great deal of anxiety around your 'forbidden' food, you need to change your thinking to, *It's just food*, the way naturally slim people think about food, even chocolate, cake, biscuits, chips, crisps, bread, ice cream, or whatever food it may be.

One of the best ways to stop all or nothing thinking is to get cognitive behavioural therapy (CBT), which teaches you to think more in grey than black-and-white terms. An example of black-and-white thinking is:

- *I need to be good and not even think about eating chocolate.*
- And after you have eaten the 'forbidden' food: *I've been 'bad', therefore I may as well give in ... and start the diet on Monday.*

To change this to more balanced thinking, you can think: *So, I've eaten a bit of chocolate. That's okay. I'm still okay.*

A study published in the *Journal of Affective Disorders* reported that when people eat to satisfy chocolate cravings, they do not crave it anymore. When chocolate was eaten for comfort, it not only prolonged depressed mood, it also made them eat more of it.[3]

Joyous path to slimness step 3: Do a trial of abstinence

Whereas it is evident from above mentioned studies that abstinence from your favourite foods makes you want them all the more, there is—as with all theories—evidence to the contrary. Look at people like Sarah Wilson who has sworn off sugar for life; look at all recovering alcoholics who will swear that abstinence is serving them much better than moderation. Different things work for different people. Thus, you could also do a trial of six months of complete abstinence from all sugar/sweets or whatever your 'forbidden food' is. After that, see if you feel better remaining abstinent. Do a trial of moderation for 6 months. If you find yourself relapsing, return to abstinence.

If you are wondering how to stop in the first place, do the ESM sequence in the 'Hyp2Hip Slimming' DVD and/or try the next few methods. I have had some of my patients prefer this complete abstinence trial whereas others do not want to be the social outcast at parties and other social functions when food is presented. Do what works for you. I've always advocated for the 'everything in moderation' model myself, but you have to find what works better for you.

Joyous path to slimness step 4: Pattern interrupt

A principle called 'pattern interrupt' may help you if you are scared of overeating on your favourite food. Pattern interrupt just means that you interrupt the usual process so that your brain begins to respond in a different way to your favourite food. For example, if you overeat chocolate, you can interrupt the pattern by eating with your left hand instead of your right hand. Or you could sit in an uncomfortable position while you are eating it, e.g. with your back to the wall, sit down as though you are sitting on a chair. Stay there while you are eating the chocolate. You will start to have negative associations with eating chocolate—you can 'rewire' your brain!

Your brain can also be rewired by changing your response to your favourite food. It involves identifying all your favourite foods. Identify one food that you can *enjoy* today. This will not be the only time you can eat it. You can eat it whenever you want. The next day eat another favourite food; the next day another one, etc. Have it, but only in moderation. If you don't think you can do this, do the 'Hyp2HipSlimming' DVD ESM exercise first.

Joyous path to slimness step 5: Find an alternative mood lift

A study has confirmed that emotional eaters have an immediate response in mood when given a palatable chocolate.[4] The researchers showed that this dependency is a conditioned response rather than due to components of the chocolate. In other words, these changes are hypothesised to occur due to the release of the feel-good hormone endorphin.[5] Further research also supports the hypothesis that the pleasure–reward system of emotional eaters is disturbed, which leads to disinhibited eating.[6] Why would you not want to eat more of what makes you feel good?

There are several things you can do to lift your mood that don't involve eating (chocolate). If you're chronically depressed, read the chapter on depression. However, if you are becoming aware that you're just depressed occasionally and find yourself eating to lift your mood, try a hobby, socialising, watching a movie, going for a walk, or doing anything that makes you feel good. Do you have enough 'play time' in your day or is it just all work?

Funny how chocolate seems to shrink clothes.

Joyous path to slimness step 6: Stop thinking, I can't have it, don't think about it

Research at the Carnegie Mellon University in Pittsburgh studied the effects of thinking about chocolate. The participants were asked to think either three or thirty times about eating chocolate M&Ms before being offered them.[7] Participants who thought about eating them thirty times ate less of them than those who thought about them only three times and those in a control condition (who imagined throwing coins into a laundry machine). What works better for you?

Part IV

Therapy Options

Chapter 12: **Hypnosis: When the Pendulum Swings, Change Begins**

'Imagination is more important than knowledge.'
(Albert Einstein)

As I have explained in the introductory chapter, the reason that *Weight Off Your Mind* is not a book about hypnosis only is because hypnosis by itself to treat eating/weight problems has not been supported much in the scientific literature. In addition, whereas hypnosis is one of the most effective methods around, it tends to work only for those who have cleared any physical/medical barriers as well as psychological blockages. Therefore, if you have skipped previous chapters, be sure to review them so that you can ensure that when you do use hypnosis, it provides you with the results you want. Furthermore, keep in mind that hypnosis is the tool to help you implement diet and exercise strategies, not a substitute for them. If you're curious about how well hypnosis can work for you:

This mesmerising chapter explains:

- ✓ What hypnosis is
- ✓ How misconceptions about hypnosis have given it a bad rap
- ✓ The evidence that hypnosis does and can work for you to achieve your weight loss goals
- ✓ Why you or other people may have failed to lose/ maintain weight with hypnosis in the past
- ✓ How to make hypnosis work for you as an adjunctive to other psychological methods

The Magic of Hypnosis—This is What Hypnosis Really Is

Getting into trance for transformation

In 1784, Franz Mesmer coined the termed 'animal magnetism' or 'mesmerism' which today is known as hypnosis.[1] What exactly is hypnosis? Some people get an idea of what hypnosis is by what they see hypnotists do on TV and thus think that being hypnotised makes people lose control and do strange things. This is stage hypnosis that aims to entertain. It shows how people can do things just by being told what to do when they believe they are in a trance state. Hypnotherapy is similar but it is used to heal rather than entertain.

The actual state of hypnosis is not an unusual state of mind at all. You are, in fact, actually hypnotised every day of your life: for example, when you wake up in the morning and remember a dream—that dreamy half-asleep state. Another example is that 'spaced out' state when you are driving a familiar route (e.g. home to work), you may get to your destination without being aware what happened in that time—that is a trance state. This trance state can by induced by someone else or you can induce yourself. Hypnotists and hypnotherapists can use a variety of different methods to induce trance. For example, a hypnotic trance induction can involve looking up, breathing, looking at a mandala, or simply by relaxation and being induced with hypnotic suggestions.

Trance is what most people think of as 'going under.' Although most people are under the impression that it is the trance that makes hypnosis work, trance has very little to do with the outcome.[2] The idea that trance is—in fact—unnecessary was also demonstrated by Ursula Markham who wrote a book *Hypnothink*. She outlines how you can hypnotise yourself just by using visualisation and hypnotic suggestions.[3]

Reason 1 hypnosis can work for you: It does not matter how hypnotisable you are.

Visualisation—the Powerhouse of Hypnosis

Apart from the trance, hypnosis also involves visualisation. A few books (including *The Gabriel Method*) have been written about the power of visualisation. Many world class sports icons including Muhammed Ali and Tiger Woods have spoken about using visualisation to succeed in their sport. World champion golfer, Jack Nicklaus has said: 'I never hit a shot, not even in practice, without having a very sharp in-focus picture of it in my head.'

Studies have actually shown that mental rehearsal of a workout is almost as effective as the real thing and that doing both is more effective than either alone. For example, investigators at the The Lerner Research Institute in Ohio investigated whether visualising doing a physical exercise was as effective as actually doing it. They found that there was a 35 percent muscle increase in the group that did the actual exercise but the visualisation-only group had a muscle increase of 13.5 percent![4] One of the things that's crucial when visualisation is used as part of hypnosis is that visualisation is more likely to work if you:

> Visualise getting through the obstacles to achieve your goal, not the goal itself.[5]

Many people worry about not getting visualisation right due to not being able to get a clear picture. The good news is that visualisation does not have to be Hollywood movie type. It will work even if you just get a vague picture. The important thing is that you have some picture of what it will look like conquering those obstacles. For example, if you know that you are going to a party full of cakes, chips, and other party foods, visualise feeling indifferent to the food and just sitting there, talking to others.

> Reason 2 hypnosis can work for you: Even just visualising yourself succeeding can work for you.

Hypnotic Suggestion—a Program to Respond

Whereas many people believe that the magic of hypnosis is in the trance or the visualisation, evidence supports that idea that hypnotic suggestion is just as important. But it is not only hypnotists who use hypnotic suggestions to make you behave in a certain way. Advertisers and sales people (especially timeshare salespeople) use hypnotic suggestions all the time. But other people including YOU may be using hypnotic suggestions without realising it. Absorbing a hypnotic suggestion is like having a CD inserted into your mind.

So, what exactly is a hypnotic suggestion? Hypnotic suggestions are statements phrased in a certain way to make you behave in a certain way. I will illustrate it with an amusing example. Many years ago, I was talking to a colleague (who was also a hypnotherapist) one day about my long bus trip home and he said to me, 'Well, whatever you do, don't fall asleep on the bus.'

I said, 'I've never fallen asleep on a bus. I won't fall asleep on the bus, don't be silly.'

But he said again, 'Just don't fall asleep on the bus.' I laughed at him, so he again repeated his statement, 'Don't fall asleep on the bus.' Well, it turns out that this particular evening, I did, in fact, fall asleep on the bus and missed my bus stop! Why? Because he had hypnotised me with the hypnotic suggestion: don't fall asleep on the bus!

This indeed—believe it or not—is a hypnotic suggestion. It's a simple (not long winded) direct statement that was potentiated by him repeating it three times and preceding it with the statement (a technique called paceing/leading) 'whatever you do'. The statement 'whatever you do' provided him with the gateway into my mind to make that happen. If he had instead said, 'If you're feeling particularly tired, don't fall asleep in the bus,' I may not have fallen asleep on the bus as I had not felt particularly tired, I responded to his suggestion 'whatever you do'. You may notice from now on how some advertisers use this art of pacing/leading and repetition. For example, you may hear a sales person say to you, 'You may think that you may never need this book. You may think someday you may need this book. But right now, as you're wondering whether to buy this book or not, you decide to buy this book.' Most people, given this hypnotic sales pitch will buy this book! This is how sly and powerful hypnosis can be.

> *'One of the most successful physicians I have ever known has assured me that he used more of bread pills, drops of coloured water, and powders of hickory ashes than of all other medicines put together.* (Thomas Jefferson)

You may not realise, but you may have been hypnotised to eat certain foods. Adverts on TV, on radio, and even logos displayed on food packaging can make you choose a certain food. The media's constant messages about having to be thin also has a tremendous power over your behaviours.[6] The case of Mr Wright's cancer cure in the 1950s illustrates exactly how much we are influenced if we don't realise that we are hypnotised.[7] According to Dr Klopfer, Mr Wright was diagnosed with lymph system cancer. At the time, the media had spread widespread news about a new miracle cure called 'Krebiozen'. Mr Wright had responded so well that his tumours had shrunk to the point that it could barely be detected. However, after reading negative reports about Krebiozen, his tumours reappeared. Believing in the power of suggestion, the doctors decided to tell Mr Wright that the batch of Krebiozen he had been given was defective and would give him the Krebiozen from a batch that was at full potency. The doctors didn't, in fact, give him any medication at all. They injected him with sterile water! Yet, Mr Wright's tumours shrank again!

A similar thing happens with other patients in hospital. When I worked at a hospital in San Diego, I was speaking to a medical resident who told me about the phenomenon of sham knee surgeries: apparently, when patients are *told* they had knee surgery after being wheeled out of the surgery room and anaesthetized, they report feeling much better even if the actual surgery is never performed! In fact, Ian Harris' book called *Surgery, the ultimate placebo* may enlighten you even more about the power of the mind.

The power of the mind was also demonstrated very well by a well-known British hypnotist Derren Brown. He did an experiment in which he gave 'a new tablet' called 'Rimoundy' to people for a variety of disorders. The result was that all of them responded favourably: their symptoms completely disappeared. It turns out he had given them a placebo (a sugar pill) and pointed out that he had scrambled 'your mind' to make up the name of the pill 'Rimoundy'.

Knowing that our minds can be influenced by what we are told, one of the most prestigious universities in the USA—Harvard Medical School—has a program in Placebo Studies & Therapeutic Encounter (PiPS). The PiPS program devotes entire studies to the phenomenon of the influence of imagination, hope, trust, persuasion, compassion, and empathic witnessing in the healing process. Throughout *Weight Off Your Mind* you will get to know how to harness the power of your mind using all of these.

The saying 'you are what you eat' is inaccurate. The truth is 'you are what you think you eat'.

But you may be surprised that this phenomenon doesn't just happen with pills. It happens with food too! To prove that it's our perception, not the actual food that influences our reaction to it, researcher Dr Crum in New York did a 'milkshake study'.[8] Now quite well known, this 'milkshake' study proved that the old saying 'you are what you eat' is very inaccurate. Participants in this 'milkshake study' were all given 380 calorie milkshakes. Half of the participants were under the impression it was a 620-calorie milkshake while the other half of participants thought it was a 140-calorie healthy shake. Those who *thought* they drank the high calorie milkshake had reduced their ghrelin levels (hunger hormone) three times more than those who thought they drank the low calorie shakes! This, again, is another piece of evidence in support of my hypothesis that most other slimming books that focus on advising you on what to eat are incomplete and that the whole point of *Weight Off Your Mind* is to change your perception of what you eat.

Indeed, our thoughts are so powerful, they influence what happens around us. Dr Masaru Emoto, author of *The Hidden Messages in Water*, shows how our thoughts, attitudes, and emotions as humans even affect our environment.[9] Dr Emoto discovered that crystals formed in frozen water when exposed to loving words shows brilliant, complex, and colourful snowflake patterns. In contrast, polluted water, or water exposed to negative thoughts, forms incomplete, asymmetrical patterns with dull colours. How this translates into weight loss is evident throughout the later chapter on social support. The gist of it as that you have the power inside your mind to change your body, your eating, and even those around you.

Reason 3 hypnosis can work for you: You can be programmed to think and behave like a slim person

Suitability and safety of hypnosis

When I did my hypnosis training in the United Kingdom in 1991, I was taught that hypnosis is suitable for almost anyone. The only exceptions are people with severe brain damage, language comprehension difficulties, and severe mental illness (e.g. psychotic disorders, severe depression). Other than that, everyone is suitable for hypnosis.

Over the past 24 years that I have been using hypnosis in clinical practice, I have never had a single incident of negative side effects. Some people, when making an appointment, have been worried about possible dangerous things that could happen during hypnosis. Rest assured, provided your hypnotherapist is properly trained and experienced:

- There's no danger of not coming out of trance
- You won't become unconscious nor is hypnosis sleep (although some people may fall asleep afterwards)
- You will be aware of everything at all times
- Your will is not weakened in any way
- You are in control and cannot be made to do anything against your will
- You will not begin to reveal information you wish to keep secret

Reason 4 hypnosis can work for you: Hypnosis is suitable for almost anyone and is safe

Hypnosis is Very Effective—See It to Believe It

When I studied psychology at university in the mid-90s, hypnosis was never taught. It wasn't even mentioned. I was made to believe that hypnosis is a form of witchcraft. It was only when I did my post-graduate studies when I did my doctoral dissertation that I received support for my interest in hypnosis. These days, hypnosis has been recognised in the National Institute for Health and Care Excellence (NICE) as a legitimate treatment. It works and it can work for you!

Although there's some research that has found treatment outcome depends on hypnotisability,[11] most research has found that it's irrelevant how hypnotisable you are.[12] The outcome depends less on how 'deep' you go and more on factors also mentioned in 'The recipe for therapy success' section in the EMDR chapter, e.g. the relationship with your therapist.[9]

Although some research has found that hypnosis is only moderately effective,[13]other researchers concluded that hypnosis is an effective tool in the treatment of obesity. They added that efficacy was improved if hypnosis was used as an adjunct to psychotherapy.[14] Another study found that when obese smokers and obese non-smokers received hypnosis-based weight loss treatment, both lost significant amounts of weight.[15]

A meta-analysis of eighteen studies investigated whether cognitive–behavioural therapy (CBT) was any better than CBT supplemented by hypnosis.[16] The researchers concluded that the addition of hypnosis substantially improved the outcome: those who had cognitive–behavioural plus hypnotherapy showed greater improvement than at least 70 percent of clients receiving CBT only treatment, particularly in the treatment of obesity. Even at long-term follow-up, those receiving hypnosis continued to lose weight after treatment ended.

In August 2005, an Australian reporter for the ABC TV science program 'Catalyst', Paul Willis, put hypnosis to the test himself for weight loss and found it easy to lose 5kg in a month. See the transcript of August 2005 'Catalyst' broadcast on 'Hypnosis'.[17]

Do you believe some things just aren't possible?

If you think eating automatically like a slim person is impossible, think about this: do you think it's possible to have an orgasm during childbirth? Apparently 0.3 percent of women do![18] At a hypnosis seminar a presenter who spoke about Hypnobirthing stated she was not only pain free during labour, she actually had an orgasm! If you can't believe it, find out more about the power of hypnosis by watching documentaries about the magic of hypnosis—it makes the impossible possible. Suggestions:

- ✓ Derren Brown: any programs at all
- ✓ On orgasmic childbirth: read *Do Birth* by Caroline Flint's or watch the documentary 'Orgasmic Birth: The Best-Kept Secret' by Debra Pascali-Bonaro.

Differences in Response to Hypnosis

Whether or not and how well you respond to hypnotic suggestions is similar to how you respond to a specific advertisement. When you buy a specific product, you may wonder why you bought that particular brand. Maybe it was because you liked the packaging or a specific ingredient not present in others; maybe you've been using it for a while and know and trust that one. But why is it that sometimes you choose one brand over another and you have no idea why? The reasons for this are the same reasons people don't buy all products that are advertised.

For example, you watch an advertisement about shampoo A. But you buy shampoo B because the ad for shampoo B evokes a stronger emotional response than shampoo A. Maybe it was because the lady who was in the ad for shampoo B is your favourite actress and you want to have hair like her. It may not be a conscious thought, but your mind recognised the expression she had on her face after she used that shampoo. In other words, it enticed the feeling of pleasure in you and your mind linked it to shampoo B. In the same way, one hypnotherapist or a particular hypnotic suggestion or visualisation will not beat the original hypnotic suggestion you already have programmed into you. But of course, there are a multitude of reasons that you won't buy a particular product: you may be worried about the cost, you may not need it, you do not know or do not trust the brand, you prefer a particular aspect of it (it is environmentally friendly or it's scientifically based), etc.

> Not responding to a particular hypnotic suggestion does not mean you aren't hypnotisable. It just means that the barrier to you changing your behaviour has not been addressed in the hypnosis.

That's why it's quite common for standard hypnotic scripts (used in commercially available hypnosis CDs or some hypnotherapists) to work for some but not for all. A standard hypnotic script for weight loss can work for most people just as an infomercial is written in such a way to address common obstacles that people have for buying a particular product. For example, a very fit and healthy looking guy will tell you how he managed to do get rock hard abs using this new ab machine. You see his six-pack and respond, *He must spend hours in the gym!* so his first line is, 'In only five minutes you can get abs like mine.' Then you think, *But I've already got a machine.* So, he tells you, 'This one is different from any other one because of features xyz.' Then you think, *I can't afford it.* So, he tells you, 'You can pay off in instalments of only $10 per week.' Then you think, *It'll be bulky, won't fit into my house.* So, he says, 'You can store it under your bed when you don't use it.' Then you think, *But I won't be motivated to do it every day.* So, he says, 'It's so easy: the machine does the work for you and you'll get a motivational video with it for free.' Then you think, *Not today. Too busy.* Then he says 'If you order today, you get a bonus: a free exercise outfit.' Thus, you buy the ab machine! You were hypnotised to buy the ab machine!

So, the infomercial has hit all the common obstacles. A standard hypnotic script usually hits all the common obstacles to weight loss but if there's even one thing that the script doesn't address—e.g. fear of too much attention—it will fail. That's the reason individualised treatment, designed specifically to you, works better. Therefore, an individual session with a hypnotherapist can address those obstacles identified during an assessment. The hypnosis used in the Hyp2Hip Slimming DVD covers a great deal of common obstacles so should do the trick—unless, as explained—you have a unique obstacle not mentioned in the script.

A patient who attended a hypnosis for weight loss session with me told me in the first session that she had a hypnosis before. She was able to quit smoking but the weight loss did not work—she had gone to the same hypnotherapist and was surprised as she had expected this therapist to get the same success with weight loss. When I did my assessment (and I always do a very thorough one), she mentioned that she was so fearful of loose skin. I said to her, 'So, if there were a 100 percent guarantee that there would be no loose skin whatsoever, would you want to lose weight?' Her answer, 'Definitely!' so we addressed this one and only obstacle. Of course, she lost weight and ... there was no loose skin!

Another lady said to me she had gone to a hypnotherapist prior to pregnancy and lost weight successfully then, but after the birth of her children had regained a few kgs. She had also returned to the same hypnotherapist seven years later but failed to lose weight. She was confused. I asked her, 'What is your barrier?' Her reply, 'If I lose weight, I can't choose where the weight comes off, so if it comes off my face, I'll look old and haggard.' Her fear of looking old and haggard was further impacted by her fear that her husband would then no longer find her attractive. Because I couldn't guarantee that she would not lose weight off her face, nor that her husband wouldn't leave her or find her unattractive, I had to work with her ability to cope with (1) not having control, and (2) being rejected for being 'unattractive'. Addressing these rather than using a standard hypnotic script is what appeared to work for her.

Path to slimness with hypnosis: make hypnosis work for you:

✓ Understand hypnosis and be open to the possibility that hypnosis can work magic on you
✓ Do the Hyp2Hip Slimming DVD
✓ Alternatively, go to www.ntpages.com.au to find a hypnotherapist in your area to get an individualised treatment
✓ Go to a hypnotherapist who is sufficiently trained and experienced and with whom you have a good therapeutic alliance

Chapter 13: **Psychological Therapy—the Diet for the Mind**

'Getting over a painful experience is much like crossing monkey bars. You have to let go at some point in order to move forward.'
(C.S. Lewis)

The Reason Psychological Therapy Can Potentiate Hypnosis

The path to your goal of achieving a happy body/weight and harmonious eating patterns can be achieved through the very powerful hypnosis method. However, if you have found that you have not yet achieved success with hypnosis, there may be psychological barriers preventing you from achieving your goals. If you have already removed the medical barriers and life barriers mentioned in the previous chapters, what are these psychological barriers that are in the way? There are many type of barriers. They include poor self-esteem, poor self-efficacy, negative associations with exercise, being slim or eating moderately, being in the habit of using food as a coping tool to deal with difficult people or situations, or associating eating certain foods (e.g. cakes, chocolate, bread, chips, etc.) with guilt and shame. These psychological barriers are, in general, not something that hypnosis can conquer. A review of the literature on hypnosis confirms its limitation in this regard. The good news is that psychological methods have been developed specifically to deal with these obstacles.

> *'The mind is its own place, and in itself can make a Heav'n of Hell, a Hell of Heav'n.'* (John Milton)

Even minor things—so called 'mini-traumas'—may be at the root of your problem. Any trauma can lead you to have poor self-esteem which in turns makes you feel unworthy, hence not giving you the strength to do things that reflect that, i.e. eating healthy or exercising regularly. In my case, for example, I experienced what is called a 'mini-trauma' which was the despair and pain I felt due to being emotionally, verbally, and—in one case—physically abused by my older brother daily for many years. For many of my patients, the trauma is either emotional or physical neglect by one or both parents (leading to the belief 'I'm not lovable') or being criticised by a caretaker, teacher, or bully (leading to the belief 'I'm not good enough').

Psychological therapy—done correctly—can resolve the psychological distress at the root of your weight and eating problem. In addition, it can undo the associations you have with food, your weight, and your shape. For us humans, food is associated with memories and associations that can be very powerful emotional cues. For example, think about how many times you have celebrated a birthday, Christmas, a wedding or other pleasant event with a dinner and/or cake. In each case, food was linked to a positive emotion. Each time you link a positive emotional experience with food, you reinforce it. You end up eating because it reminds you of positive emotions and/or removes any negative emotions you may have. You may notice that you eat more during times of stress, during depression, or when you are feeling an uncomfortable emotion.

Life begins at the end of your comfort zone

Many people aren't aware how potent psychological therapy can be. However, research has shown—for example—that when psychotherapy is compared to treatment with medication, psychotherapy can be equally as effective. For example, when Cognitive Behavioural Therapy (CBT) was compared to anti-depressant medication, CBT was found to have as much effect on the physiology as anti-depressant medication.[1]

To achieve your weight and eating goal, change the way you think about food, your body, and your weight. Then it is easy to maintain it. Psychological therapy can help you with this.

The Effectiveness of Psychological Therapy: The Proof is in the Pudding

Diet and exercise programs need to have a psychological component to make them work

An analysis of thirty-seven studies, representing over 16,000 overweight and obese adult participants, found that greater weight loss was associated with the combination of calorie counting, contact with a dietitian, and use of psychological methods (behaviour change techniques).[2] Another major study of thirty-six randomised controlled trials involving 3,495 patients was included in a study that showed behavioural therapy (as a stand-alone treatment) was associated with greater reductions in weight (a loss of 2.5kg–3.3kg) compared with placebo.[3] However, when behavioural therapy was combined with diet or exercise interventions, then compared with diet and exercise in combination, the intervention that incorporated behavioural therapy resulted in a greater weight reduction. Increasing the intensity of the behavioural intervention significantly increased weight loss (change in weight of –2.3 kg to –3.3 kg). Cognitive–behavioural therapy, when combined with a diet and exercise intervention, resulted in greater weight loss than diet or exercise alone (–4.9kg to –2.4 kg).

Psychological therapy has been proven to eliminate binge eating

A major study, which reviewed a total of thirty-eight studies with 1973 participants, found that cognitive behavioural-based psychotherapy and structured self-help are effective in reducing binge eating.[4] Although different types of psychological therapies have varying outcomes, most have shown that psychological therapies in general are very effective. For example, a study published in *Archives of General Psychiatry* compared 205 women and men with a body mass index (BMI) of 27–45 who met criteria for Binge Eating Disorder (BED) who underwent twenty sessions of interpersonal psychotherapy (IPT) or behavioural weight loss treatment (BWL) or ten sessions of cognitive behaviour therapy-based guided self-help. A two-year follow-up, the IPT and

CBT-guided self-help were more effective in helping people stop binge eating than BWL.[5]

Psychological therapies have a high success rate with treating BED

In 1995, the *American Psychologist* journal published an article about a *Consumer Reports* survey of 4,000 people who had received psychotherapy. The results indicated that 54 percent said psychotherapy helped 'a great deal' and 90 percent reported it helped at least 'somewhat'.[6] Different types of therapies have different results. A study comparing cognitive behaviour therapy (CBT) with behavioural weight loss (BWL) found that 67 percent of those in the CBT group and 47 percent of the BWL group had a 70 percent reduction in binge eating by week four.

Although more CBT participants reduced binge eating (compared to the BWL), they didn't achieve weight loss. However, whereas the BWL participants had lower rates of reduction in binge eating, they achieved short-term weight loss. One of the other interesting finding in this study was that 62 percent of those who responded rapidly, stopped binge-eating compared to 13 percent for the slow responders. Quick responders had greater reductions in binge-eating frequency, but also had greater reduction in the severity of eating disorder symptoms and more weight loss. Those without rapid response failed to improve further.[7]

Self-help works but attending therapy is best

Research published in the *American Journal of Psychiatry* investigated whether self-help group treatment could be as effective as therapy-assisted and therapist led therapy.[8] A total of 259 adults diagnosed with Binge Eating Disorder (BED) were assigned to either 20 weeks of therapist-led; therapist-assisted; self-help group treatment; or no treatment. After treatment, the therapist-led group had the best result with an abstinence rate of 51 percent. Although much better than the participants who had no treatment (with an abstinence rate of 10 percent), the therapist-assisted group had an abstinence rate of only a 33 percent and the self-help had only 17 percent. The therapist-led condition also showed more reductions in binge eating at end of treatment and follow-up assessments compared to those who received self-help.

Although some people report benefitting from self-help books, it seems—at least from the above evidence—that attending therapy is best. To find a psychologist in Australia, you can go to www.psychology.org.au, then click on Find a Psychologist, then enter your details: adult, weight management or body image, and postcode and you should be able to find a psychologist in your area. Or you can get a referral to a psychologist (working in the field of eating disorder, body image problems, or weight management problems) from your GP.

Also consider my 'Weight Off Your Mind' workshops (see www.weightoffyourmind.net).

What is cognitive behavioural therapy (CBT)?

Cognitive Behaviour Therapy is a type of psychological therapy that aims to help you to think and perceive things differently. Epictetus said, 'What upsets people is not things themselves but their judgments about the things.' CBT is all about changing unhelpful thoughts and beliefs about food, dieting, shape, weight, and self-contempt and can assist in curbing overeating and binge eating,

For example, you may have an irrational belief about food, e.g. 'eating helps me cope'. The consequence of this belief is that you have an irresistible urge to eat especially in times when you believe you're not coping with things. The CBT-psychologist can assist you with techniques (the cognitive change) to help you believe alternative beliefs, e.g. 'food is just food. It is relieves hunger only. In fact, it causes me more grief if I eat too much'.

The behavioural part would be to find things to do that help you cope with so called 'coping actions'. For example, you will be more motivated to engage in behaviours such as exercising or distracting yourself from the urge to eat by talking to a friend or doing breathing exercises instead of (binge) eating to calm down.

CBT has been practiced widely for more than 30 years. It has been researched extensively, and has been found to be effective with a variety of emotional psychological difficulties.[9] Other psychological therapies have recently emerged: mindfulness based cognitive therapy (MBCT), acceptance and commitment therapy (ACT), dialectical behaviour therapy (DBT), and schema therapy.

What is behaviour/behavioural therapy?

Unlike psychodynamic or psychoanalytic therapies that uncover childhood issues, behavioural therapy focuses on changing current behaviour directly. Behavioural therapy is based on the theory of classical conditioning and operant conditioning such as positive and negative reinforcements, punishment as well as extinction. This means that all behaviours, including eating behaviour, are learned. Because a behaviour is learned, it can be unlearned. This means, for example, that if you associate food with reward or relaxation, it's because you may have had frequent association or a major association with these reinforcers (rewards) at some point in your life. For example, if your parents rewarded your good behaviour by buying you chocolate, you will tend to associate chocolate with something positive.

Behaviour therapies use short-term approaches such as aversion therapy, systematic desensitisation, and flooding/exposure therapy. Aversion therapy involves techniques that 'puts you off' whichever food you find irresistible. Desensitisation, a more gradual (but less time efficient) form of flooding, involves exposing you to a particular stimulus (e.g. chocolate) until you no longer react to it (i.e. react with the urge to have to eat it).

Psychological therapy works but you need enough of it

Although I would like to say that in all the years I have been in clinical practice, I've had 100 percent success, this is simply not the case. I, like every therapist, haven't been able to help every single person who was in therapy with me. There are many things that make therapy work and some things that prevent it from working: therapist characteristics, the type of therapy, the therapeutic relationship, as well as your own circumstances all affect the outcome. In addition, if you don't get enough therapy, you are unlikely to get a successful outcome. Going to therapy for a few sessions without completing treatment is the same as taking antibiotics for a few days rather than taking the full course. It's simply not effective enough.

I have had some people come to therapy asking, 'How much is enough therapy?' fearing that they need to be in therapy for years. Fortunately, in most cases, therapy does not take years. Whereas it does depend on the complexity of your problem; eating disorder experts have concluded that standard cognitive behavioural therapy for Binge Eating Disorder is best delivered over a course of twenty-two sessions in six months.[10]

I would agree with the research evidence that the more sessions, the better the outcome. Research has found that long term therapy is particularly helpful as initial changes in the brain are just temporary. Thus, the longer the therapy, the more the memory or nerve pathways get reinforced.[11] In my practice, most people who have come to me for binge eating and weight problems have come with a multitude of other problems, mostly a history of sexual abuse and have thus needed many more sessions, usually at least ten.

However, I have also seen excellent results of people coming for only one or two sessions! So, how do you know if you need only one or two sessions? Looking at the patients who needed only one or two sessions, the following were my observations—short term therapy was successful for those who were:

- Highly motivated,
- Did not have another major mental health problem (e.g. a mood or anxiety disorder),
- Were not overly stressed about any other aspect in their lives (e.g. relationships, financial, relocation, etc.)
- Did not have a family history of obesity
- Did not have a long history of binge eating and/or weight management problems
- Responded to EMDR (a type of psychological therapy described in the next chapter)

How many sessions will you need? Unfortunately, there is no straight answer to this. My recommendation is to stay in therapy for as long as you need to, which is when both you and the therapist agree that you have reached your goals. A major mistake is to leave therapy when it gets 'too hard'.

Apart from actual therapy duration, the length of an actual therapy session also appears to make a difference. According to Dr Matthew Bambling of the Neurobiology of Behavioral Change, a therapist and client become physiologically aligned (through the nervous system) during a therapy session.[12] Consequently, the better the relationship, the better the response, i.e. your therapist will impact your brain just by being there! Ideal alignment occurs with 90-120 minute sessions. Unfortunately, most therapists (especially psychologists) offer only 50-60 minute sessions. This is mostly because the majority of therapists have been taught that a therapy session is an hour long. It's also because in Australia, Medicare-funded therapy supports the conventional hour long therapy period. If you find a therapist who offers 90 minute sessions, go with that.

Therapy can be affordable

As noted above, psychological therapies have solid scientific evidence for their efficacy as a treatment for your eating and weight problem. If you have financial concerns, there are several options. In Australia, you are likely to be eligible to get a Mental Health Care Plan, which can be obtained by making an appointment with a G.P. and requesting a referral to a psychologist. Currently, this Mental Health Care Plan will entitle you to ten sessions per year that attracts a significant Medicare rebate (i.e. up to $124.50 rebate per session for a clinical psychologist). Some psychologists bulk bill, which means you wouldn't have to pay a gap.

Alternatively, if you have private health care, check with them to see how much psychological therapy is covered. Or, if you work for a company that offers Employee Assistance Programs (EAP), you can make an appointment there. Bear in mind that most EAP providers offer only five to six sessions per year. Also ensure that the therapist at the EAP service is suitably qualified and experienced in the Binge Eating Disorder field.

Finally, another way to save costs is to take group rather than individual therapy. Although some studies have shown that individual therapy is superior to group therapy,[13] other research has not confirmed this.[14] In my clinical experience, group therapy is very effective. If all else fails and you have to pay for therapy privately, think of it as an investment in yourself. Rather than saving up for a holiday, save up for therapy.

Summary of psychological therapy—the diet for the mind

- ✓ You are more likely to overcome your eating and weight problems if you combine diet and exercise programs with a psychological intervention
- ✓ Done correctly, psychological therapy can remove the underlying cause of your problematic eating and eliminate the urge to eat to cope with problems and hence enhance hypnosis
- ✓ A variety of different psychological therapies are available (CBT, behavioural therapy, interpersonal therapy, etc.) and offer an affordable way to help you quit binge eating. EMDR is a very powerful method (see next chapter)
- ✓ You are more likely to accelerate the effect of hypnosis if you attend psychological therapy with a qualified, experienced psychologist (more so than simply using self-help books)

Chapter 14: **EMDR and Alternative Methods**

'Do just once what others say you cannot do and you will never pay attention to their limitations again.'
(Captain James Cook)

EMDR: Weight Loss in the Blink of an Eye

When I began my studies in psychology in 1993, I was taught psychodynamic and psychoanalytic therapies, but the majority of my training was in a type of therapy called cognitive behaviour therapy (CBT) because it is the one 'evidence-based' treatment that has received a great deal of research support. For Binge Eating Disorder—according to scientific literature—CBT too is still considered the gold class.[1] However, in my own clinical experience with hundreds of people since 2001, I have found hypnosis, ESM, and the psychological treatment called Eye Movement Desensitisation Reprocessing (EMDR) to be the quickest and most effective therapies. But I am not alone. As mentioned, hypnosis is not the crux of *Weight Off Your Mind*, not because hypnosis doesn't work. Hypnosis definitely works but not without removing the physical, life, and also the mind barriers so that the power of hypnosis can do all the work for you. I will explain in this chapter how a unique psychological therapy called EMDR can remove the 'mind barriers'.

EMDR, or Eye Movement Desensitisation Reprocessing, is a method that was created by psychologist Dr Francine Shapiro in 1987.[2] It was originally used only for the treatment of trauma/post traumatic stress disorder (PTSD) related to sexual/physical abuse or combat but since then has been applied to many other disorders including panic attacks, phobias, grief, pain, addictions, as well as eating disorders. Researchers are still investigating how it works. Currently, EMDR is explained through the 'adaptive information processing' (AIP) model: when a person has an upsetting experience, the brain is unable to process this properly. The moment becomes 'frozen in time' so that a person continues to experience the same event long after its occurrence due to being triggered by sounds, smells, images, and feelings about the event. EMDR allows the information to be processed in such a way as to desensitise the person: this means the memory of the upsetting event can be remembered; however, the emotions will be cleared.

In practice what this means is that you will be able to remember the traumatic experience but you won't have the accompanying emotional response—it's as though it happened to someone else, not you. EMDR appears to have a similar process to REM (rapid eye movement) sleep. It's thus considered a more physiologically based therapy. Unlike regular psychotherapy sessions in which the therapist elicits the person to talk in detail about the traumatic event, EMDR does not require this. The upsetting event is brought to mind only very briefly. It is then processed by bilateral eye movements that are facilitated by the therapist who guides the person's eyes for up to one minute at a time. The sequence is repeated until the distress about the event has cleared. What makes EMDR work is not so much the eye movements themselves (as it can also be done with auditory or kinaesthetic stimulation), but how and what is processed during those eye movements. Thus, it takes a trained, skilled, experienced therapist (not just a computer image) to complete an EMDR session. That's why the EMDR sessions you can access over the internet are unlikely to be effective.

So, EMDR is the perfect method to eliminate binge eating and/or weight/body image problems when a trauma is at the root of it. However, if you're thinking you don't have anything in the past that was 'traumatic', rest assured. The definition of 'trauma' encompasses not only what is traditionally considered a 'trauma'. Thus, even if you haven't experienced sexual or physical abuse or seen someone die in front of you, for example, EMDR is still applicable. The reason is that in EMDR, a 'trauma' is considered to be anything that you may have experienced as emotionally overwhelming. For example, did you witness your parents fighting, then divorcing? Did you blame yourself? Did you lose your best friend when your family moved? Were you bullied at school or by a sibling? Did you feel unloved or abandoned when your parents 'abandoned' you by going to work? Did you experience grief when your grandmother died or when your spouse left you? All this is considered trauma.

The number of sessions required vary from person to person and also varies depending on the nature and complexity of the problem. Some people may need only one session for a particular problem whereas others may find they need three, six, or ten or more sessions. Typically, a single event trauma is cleared in one session whereas traumatic events that occurred repeatedly over many years require at least three sessions. EMDR is known for its efficiency—compared to more lengthy treatments like psycho-analytic therapies, which can take years.

The Evidence That EMDR Works

Dr Shapiro's initial findings of being able to treat trauma were published in the *Journal of Traumatic Stress* in 1989. Since then thousands of research papers and books have been written. *The Journal of EMDR Practice and Research* was first published in July 2007. Whereas thousands of researchers have focused their research on PTSD (trauma) treatment, more recent research has investigated the efficacy of EMDR on many other disorders including binge eating.

If you are interested in reading the research, go to the websites:

www.emdraa.org
www.emdria.org
www.emdr.com

Many official agencies around the world have recommended EMDR as a treatment of choice for trauma:[3]

- The Substance Abuse and Mental Health Services Administration (SAMHSA) is an agency of the U.S. Department of Health and Human Services (HHS). This national registry (NREPP) cites EMDR as evidence based practice for treatment of PTSD, anxiety, and depression
- EMDR is a treatment listed for PTSD in the Therapy Advisor (2004-7) which lists only empirically supported methods

- EMDR was placed in the 'A' category (strongly recommended) for the treatment of trauma in the Department of Veterans Affairs & Department of Defense (2004)
- EMDR is a designated treatment of choice for PTSD in the UK, Netherlands, and France.
- EMDR was stated to be an empirically supported treatment for adult PTSD in the National Institute for Clinical Excellence (2005). Post-traumatic stress disorder (PTSD): The management of adults and children in primary and secondary care. London: NICE Guidelines.

Because it so highly regarded, EMDR is a widely practiced therapy: worldwide over 70,000 practitioners practice it, mostly in Europe and the USA. Some weight loss boot camps in the USA offer EMDR sessions. Unfortunately, there are not many EMDR practitioners in Australia and you are likely to find it difficult to find an EMDR therapist in Australia who is familiar with using it to treat Binge Eating Disorder, as most of them are trained to treat primarily the trauma disorder PTSD with it. However, if you do find an EMDR practitioner you may still find it beneficial for your issues as it can help you overcome the underlying traumas.

To find an EMDR practitioner, go to www.emdr.com.au or www.emdria.com. I personally trained two psychologists in 2014 in Sydney and do not know of any other therapists who are trained or experienced to apply EMDR to Binge Eating Disorder (BED). However, if you do have an opportunity to go to an experienced EMDR therapist to help you achieve your weight loss goal, please look into it. Please also consider my 'Weight Off Your Mind' workshops (see www.weightoffyourmind.net). The application of EMDR for Binge Eating Disorder, at the moment, is limited to my research at the University of Sydney as well two other people who presented at EMDR conferences in Italy[4] and Belgium.[5]

In other words, whereas EMDR is a perfect choice, to date there's not enough scientific evidence to support its use for the treatment of weight/body image problems and Binge Eating Disorder (BED). I have no doubt that it works, but as stated above, finding a therapist who is experienced to use it for BED may be a challenge. Fortunately, I have a solution for this. One option is to attend my 'Weight Off Your Mind' workshops. The second option is to simply use any of the evidence-based psychological therapies mentioned in the previous chapter. The other option to air out your fat is to use the alternative method called breathwork.

> *'If you have enough butter, anything is good.'* (Julia Child)

Breathwork—Breathe a Sigh of Relief if All Else Has Failed

According to the Breathwork Association Australia, breathwork is a form of therapy that helps to resolve issues, dissolve limiting decisions, and release unhealthy attachment to past events. It can also assist you to achieve your full potential, generating a feeling of aliveness and sense of inspiration. It achieves this through awareness and experience of the breath, which creates balance and a sense of wellbeing and purpose. At the end of a session, you may feel more positive about life or even have an entirely new perspective.[6]

According to Dr Andrew Weil[1], a proponent of breathwork, 'there's no single more powerful—or more simple—daily practice to further your health and well-being than Breathwork.'[7] The way breathwork was explained to me when I was in a course that included Holotropic Breathwork exercise was that the hyperventilation also detoxes and rejuvenates. In the 45-minute session, I had a very profound experience as I felt like I was releasing past mini-trauma. I was in a group with about ninety-six other people all of whom said they either had a full body orgasm, had a spiritual experience, or like me had uncontrollable laughter. This was, however, preceded by crying. Some people were also crying but also had diarrhoea, vomited, or became temporarily semi-unconscious. It was explained to me that the unconsciousness was due to detoxing from previous anaesthetics—hence, the more anaesthetics you've had, the more often you experience these semi-unconscious states. Most (like me) didn't actually know why we were crying or laughing, whereas some identified events, e.g. being told by a parent 'you're no good'.

Whether or not having such an experience benefited me, I don't know. Although I experienced some positive changes following this breathwork exercise; it's unclear whether I could attribute it to the breathwork itself or the other things I did to achieve my goals. However, I certainly enjoyed the laughter. Based on a study of more than 11,000 people doing Holotropic Breathing over more than twelve years, breathwork has no adverse side effects and is thus

---

[1] Dr Weil is author of seven books on mind/body healing, director of the Program in Integrative Medicine and clinical professor of Internal Medicine at the University of Arizona at Tucson, USA.

considered a low risk therapy.[8] Thus, at the very least, you'll have a good time doing breathwork, and at the worst, you will have no effect at all.

Whereas I cannot guarantee that breathwork will help you achieve your weight management goal, I believe it's worth trying. If you're wondering why I would suggest a method that is not scientifically-based as a potential alternative to EMDR, it is because I have personally experienced this method and feel that, even if it's merely a placebo-effect, it has the potential to unlock something that regular psychological therapy may not. Nevertheless, my recommendation remains the same: first do psychological therapy (EMDR if available) followed by hypnosis; if psychological therapy has not worked for you (or if EMDR is not available), then try breathwork. See more on www.australianbreathworkassociation.org.au or find a practitioner on ntpages.com.au. The only other alternative method I suggest are the meridian stimulation methods described below.

Tapping Into the Power of Meridian Stimulation

In the preface I mentioned that I had been trained in 2001 in ESM (Emotional Self-Management) by well-respected psychologists and founders of the ESM method Dr Pratt and Dr Lambrou in San Diego. A variation of the more commonly known method Thought Field Therapy (TFT), it involves tapping meridian points, saying affirmations, and doing various eye movements. Researchers are still trying to investigate why it works, but so far have identified that stimulating meridian points releases serotonin (the feel good chemical) in parts of the brain.[9]

For some time after I did the ESM course, I used it almost exclusively as I had excellent results. After about two years, I hardly using it not only because I found that EMDR and hypnosis were more efficient, but also because people thought ESM was weird. Neither does ESM have scientific evidence. However, I did meet a girl who reported great benefits from ESM treatment for the trauma she had after being kidnapped by the Mexican Mafia. In addition, my trainers Dr Lambrou and Pratt, both very well respected psychologists in San Diego, cited many success stories. The beauty of ESM also is that it can be done without having to go to a therapist. Given all of these positive indications of the power of ESM, I have included the ESM component in the Hyp2Hip Slimming DVD.

Whereas ESM doesn't have scientific support, other versions of it have found some support. The original Thought Field Therapy (TFT), developed by psychologist Roger Callahan, is based on the theory that emotional disturbances can be resolved by stimulating meridian points.[10] Callahan published a book *The Five Minute Phobia Cure* and claims to be able to treat a variety of mental health problems with TFT. Since then, other forms of TFT have been developed. The Emotional Freedom Technique (EFT) was developed by Gary Craig in 2001.[11] Based on Thought Field Therapy (TFT), he believed by using a comprehensive tapping sequence, it eliminates the need to identify a specific sequence, thus making it a less of a 'hit or miss' method.

Like all alternative therapies, TFT has not been researched extensively. However, one study showed that 103 of the 105 people who had been treated with TFT for war trauma reported an absence of trauma symptoms, even five months after treatment.[12] However, this study was heavily criticised for not adhering to normal research protocols. In terms of binge eating and weight management, EFT is slowly showing promise as research of its efficacy is emerging. For example, Dr Peta Stapleton at Queensland's Griffith University School of Medicine has done some research on the efficacy of Emotional Freedom Technique (EFT). I attended a seminar at the Eating Disorders and Obesity conference in 2014 in which she presented her research on EFT. Her research found EFT to be helpful in eliminating food cravings or 'willpower over food'.[13]

Based on this evidence, I would recommend doing the ESM exercises on the Hyp2Hip Slimming DVD. Alternatively, if you would like to attend sessions with a practitioner in person, you may find one on www.ntpages.com.au. Given the fact that both breathwork and Though Field Therapy-based methods are so unconventional, I would recommend the following guidelines to ensure that the therapist you choose is suitable/appropriate.

3 Ingredients for Therapy Success

1. Treatment works best when you have a good relationship with your practitioner

A large body of research has provided evidence that it doesn't matter so much what type of treatment is used, it's the therapeutic alliance that makes treatment work.[14] Thus, the need to go to a treatment with someone with whom you have a good relationship applies to any therapy—whether it is a GP, psychologist, dietitian, or alternative therapist. Having rapport with a therapist means you trust him or her and get along. Good rapport and a good working relationship is likely to be established if:

- The therapist clarifies what happens in therapy in a particular session, including clarifying expectations
- Sets mutually acceptable goals
- Begins and ends sessions on time and uses time effectively (avoids chit-chat, doesn't go overtime or finish early)
- Remains respectful, empathic, understanding, compassionate, and non-judgmental
- Clarifies your responsibilities
- Ends therapy when it is no longer necessary
- Is open to feedback from you when you feel you are not moving forward
- Keeps your details strictly confidential
- Is ethical and professional
- Makes you feel comfortable but still pushes you beyond your comfort zones
- Allows you to see things from a new perspective that brings about changes you want

If you notice that a particular practitioner dismisses your weight management concerns with a comment that indicates that he or she does not understand your distress, it means this particular practitioner is not suitable for you. If you are concerned about your weight and/or your eating, so should a health practitioner. A pleasant 'bedside manner' is very important when you don't want to be told to just 'wire your mouth shut' or 'just eat less and exercise more' or 'you look fine. Just don't worry about it'.

Remember that your therapist should not be your friend. Your therapist should be gentle but have enough strength to push you beyond your comfort zones. You will have to share a great deal of personal information (and the therapist should not share theirs unless it is relevant) and may expose you to things you don't want to talk about. It is painful—in some cases—so, apart from a box of tissues—the therapist also needs to be able to have a strong enough relationship with you to get you to the place in which you feel safe to address all of it.

2. Find a therapist with the best qualifications, education, and experience

The scientific research has supported the evidence that the more qualified and experienced the therapist, the better the outcome.[15] This may be partly due to the fact that the more experienced a therapist, the more confident the therapist. Someone who has gone to university for six to eight years is likely to be more enthusiastic about therapy compared to someone who has gone to university only four years. I am not implying that all therapists who have only a certificate, diploma, or bachelor's degree are not as good as someone with a Masters or Doctorate degree though. Other factors affect the outcome of the therapy. However, overall, ideally your search should be focused on finding a therapist with the highest qualifications and most experience in dealing with your particular problems.

Choosing the right therapist appears to be so important that an effective physician giving you a placebo can achieve better results than a poor physician using an effective psychoactive agent.[16]

3. Go to a therapist who practices what he/she preaches

The psychology research supports the evidence that a good therapist is one who is sufficiently qualified and experienced but also mentally healthy to be in a position to help. There are sometimes very well meaning therapists out there wanting to help but really should not. They may still be struggling with their own issues and may have taken a course to help themselves rather than others. They may fail to apply the principles they teach to their patients to themselves. Then there are those—probably not many—who do a weekend course in a therapy (typically hypnosis) and believe they are qualified to practice simply because they have a certification. The therapist's health and skill as well as interest in helping people determine whether you will get better. [17]

How do you know whether he or she is healthy enough to help you? It's not easy when you are looking online or in a phone book and read about a therapist's qualifications. With weight and eating, it's—to some extent—easier to figure out: some therapists are overweight and obese themselves (although this does not necessarily mean they struggle with binge eating). The question to ask though is whether you would you trust him or her to do therapy on you. Other things to watch out for may be how the therapist sounds on the phone, how the practice is set up, and how the therapist presents themselves. If your impressions of those things is that you don't admire them or don't feel comfortable at the first session, then you're unlikely to establish a good relationship.

Part V

Putting It All Together

Chapter 15: **What to Eat to Slim Down**

'Let food be thy medicine.'
(Hippocrates)

Do 'Diets' Work?

If you are like many people who have had battles with their eating and/or weight, you are likely to have been on diet after diet and find it unsustainable, too expensive, boring, or making you constantly think about food. Patients who have come to my office complain about the fact that most diets don't teach them a new lifestyle or a behaviour. Diets are all about restrictions: you must eat this, must not eat that. So, if a 'diet' isn't the answer, what do you need to eat to slim down and stay slim?

I recently saw a book entitled *Lose weight without dieting or working out. Interesting*, I thought—no diet or exercise needed. When I had a look at its contents, I discovered it was written by a nutritionist who advocated eating 'clean foods' and encouraged 'physical activity'. In other words: diet and exercise! Is there a way around it? We know that the diet and exercise strategy is what to do—but how to do it is very often not revealed in weight loss success stories. Fortunately, as you read, knowing that you have now eliminated all the barriers to making hypnosis work for you, it's time now to find out exactly what to eat.

Look at the evidence of what works: whereas in 2008 singer Ricki-Lee Coulter apparently 'embraced her curves', she went on to lose 30kg (going from size 14 to size 8) by cutting out potatoes, dairy, bread, and other wheat products. While still allowing herself to have the odd treat of chocolate, pizza, dessert, and alcohol in moderation, she reportedly goes for 1-hour runs 5-6 mornings a week.[1] Kate Ritchie apparently lost weight to slim down for her wedding by exercising and working on portion control.[2] Kerri-Anne Kennerley also lost 8kg (a dress size) with the help of her Dancing with the Stars' dancing partner Carmelo, who not only trained 6 hours a day with her at some stage, but also recommended changing her diet, which included portion control.[3] Former 'Sunrise' presenter Melissa Doyle lost 10kg (two dress sizes) in 2013 by exercising 30-minutes per day and eating healthier, although she reportedly didn't go on a 'diet' as such. With three meals a day and no snacking on sweets, she's maintained her weight.[4] Comedienne Julia Morris lost 20kg (size 16 to 12) in 18 months, reportedly avoiding all carbohydrates after 5pm, having three meals a day and no snacks, cutting out all added sugar and working out with the help of a personal trainer twice weekly.[5]

This diet + exercise strategy is echoed in the scientific literature. A report in the *British Medical Journal of a* systematic review of 45 trials involving 7,788 people confirmed that exercise and diet (change in eating) is beneficial for weight loss and maintenance.[9] Another study supporting the diet + exercise intervention was supported by a systematic review of 80 studies of weight-loss interventions leading to successful outcomes found that the average weight loss was 5 to 8.5kg during the first 6 months from interventions involving a reduced-energy diet and/or weight-loss medications with weight plateaus at approximately 6 months. After 4 years, the average weight loss was 3 to 6kg, which was maintained with none experiencing weight regain to baseline. Compared to the diet-exercise combination, exercise-only groups experienced minimal weight loss at any time point.[7]Another systematic review of thirty-three clinical trials investigating diet and exercise showed this combination was effective even for one year follow up.[8] No surprise, but more specifically, another article published in the *American Journal of Clinical Nutrition* found that maintainers do the following:[9]

- Exercise about one hour a day
- Eat a low-calorie, low-fat diet
- Eat breakfast regularly
- Have a consistent eating pattern across weekdays and weekends

None of the weight loss success stories about Ricki-Lee, Kate, KAK, Mel, and Lady Julia, nor the scientific literature, explain how they were able to do this but all have a similar story: they have all adjusted their diet and added exercise. I too lost weight by eating more salads, eating fewer meals with rich sauce, reducing sugar intake, and of course, no longer binge eating. These ladies spoke about what they did to lose and maintain their weight, not how they did it or that it was easy or difficult. Fortunately, that's where hypnosis fits in beautifully, as it makes the journey much easier than white-knuckling through it.

With so much misinformation about diets out there, I won't blame you if you have—like so many chronic dieters—lost touch with your own hunger and are completely confused as to what to eat and what not to eat. One diet says 'eat wholemeal bread', another says 'don't eat any grains at all'; one diet says 'low carb is the way', another says, 'you need carbs to boost your mood'. So, who is right? To answer that question, here are some facts according to the obesity guidelines published in the *Obesity Journal* (2014)[10]:

- There isn't one particular diet that is superior but a diet that creates a calorie deficit is recommended
- The diet must be one that a person can stick to in the long term and
- The diet must be nutritionally balanced

Furthermore:

- The *New England Journal of Medicine* reported a study that compared different types of diets. Researchers found that success did not depend on the type of diet—success was dependent on whether dieters could stick to a diet[11]
- Similarly, a study of the Atkins diet (low carb), The Zone ('anti-inflammatory' good fat diet), Weight Watchers, and Ornish plans (low fat diet) noted that all had similar weight loss, but noted that adherence to the diet made a difference[12]
- Researchers at the University of Kansas Medical Center found that of 179 participants, 76.5 percent had successfully maintained their weight loss of at least 5 percent. One of their conclusions was that maintainers were those who were able to reduce the level of perceived effort required for long-term weight control[13]

- Another study of 931 participants published in *Obesity Research* (2000) found the same result[14]
- Prominent eating disorder researcher Dr Marsha Marcus of the Western Psychiatric Institute and Clinic in Pittsburgh recommends a program that identifies a regular eating plan, not one with 'diet rules'[15] This means any diet that excludes a particular food type or has rules as to when and what you can eat, is bound to fail.

'The second day of a diet is always easier than the first: by the second day, you're off it.' (Jackie Gleason)

The thing about diets is that different people react differently to the same diet. For example, a study called *POUNDS Lost* found similar weight loss, regardless of the type of diet. However, they found that some people lost over 20kg and others actually gained weight on the diets. They concluded that it boiled down to our genes, identifying eleven different genes predictive of response.[16]

In this study of 177,330 individuals in forty studies in eight-five centres around the world, researchers concluded that individuals with a certain genotype respond better than those without this genotype by choosing a high-carbohydrate and low-fat diet.[17] Hence, the reason that some people do really well on a low carbohydrate diet whereas others actually gain weight on this type of diet. At this point, unless you want to get a genetic test, it may just be a matter of trial and error to figure out what works for you. However, as mentioned above, a low calorie diet appears to be the best option anyway.

'If one doesn't have the character like Abraham Lincoln or Joan of Arc, a diet is simply disintegrates into eating exactly what you want to eat, but with a bad conscience.' (Maria Augusta Trapp)

In sum: forget the idea there is one diet that works for everyone and therefore should work for you. Figure out what works for you. Bear in mind above advice (and recommendation throughout *Weight Off Your Mind*) that the diet you choose should be one that provides you with all the nutrition you need and be easy to sustain. You have the power of hypnosis right behind you so that you can bypass your emotional brain and respond to logical hypnotic suggestions, e.g. eat low calorie foods. The following is an outline of different types of low calorie diets:

The Low Calorie Diet

When I was growing up in the 1980s, low calorie diets were all the rage. In Germany, we had a saying 'FDH' ('Friss die Haelfte') which translates to 'eat half'. Imagine how much weight you could lose if you 'just ate half' of what you have been eaten. It's actually easier than you think—as long as you have some awareness of calories.

I had a patient attend therapy who stated that she couldn't understand why she wasn't losing weight: she said she neither grazes, nor eats junk food, nor eats too much. She didn't exercise, but I didn't believe lack of activity was the major problem. Her GP had ruled out any medical problems, so I sent her to a dietitian just to check her diet. The dietitian confirmed that her diet was indeed rather healthy, but her portion sizes were just too big. Even though she believed she 'doesn't eat that much', the dietitian explained to her that she was actually eating way too much by explaining to her what a serving size is: e.g. 50g of chicken or the size of a palm; 1 serving of tuna is about 50g (¼ tin); 1 serving of yoghurt is 285g, a serving of cheese the size of a matchbox, etc. Only then did she realise that she was actually eating too much: her portion sizes were double of what she was supposed to eat—hence doubling her calorie intake. No wonder she wasn't losing weight.

As you have read above, as per the Obesity Guidelines, a low calorie diet is the recommended diet. According to research conducted at the National Weight Control Registry (with 355 women and 83 men who had maintained a weight loss of at least 13.6kg for at least 1 year or had lost an average of 30kg and maintained the weight loss for 5.1 years), they all continued consumption of a low-energy and low-fat diet. For women a low calorie diet is about 1,306 calories per day with 24 percent of energy from fat and men about 1,685 kcal with 23 percent of energy from fat.[18] A systematic review of fourteen randomised controlled trials found that low fat, 600 calorie deficit, or low calorie diets were associated with weight loss of about 5kg at 12 months.[19] Although this may not appear to be much weight, remember that this was a diet-only intervention that did not include exercise, psychological methods, nor addressing medical issues. The thing to keep in mind if you choose a low calorie diet are:

- Due to metabolism decreases, exercise is recommended to counteract this[20]
- To minimise muscle loss, ensure that you have at least 60 grams (or 0.8–1.5g per kg) of protein[21]

- Since low calorie diets tend to make you lose a great deal of water, particularly in the first week,[22] don't get disheartened if you don't lose as much weight later on in the diet. Just because you're not losing as much weight as before, it doesn't necessarily mean you're not losing cms or fat—so it's still best to measure yourself with a tape measure and to use a scale that measures body fat and muscle rather than just weight

'Food is an important part of a balanced diet.'
(Fran Lebowitz)

Dietitian's Advice for Weight Loss

If you like the idea 'everything in moderation', then you will like what dietitians have to say. I would recommend having at least one session with a dietitian, especially if you are vegetarian, are Celiac, or have food allergies, intolerances, sensitivities, or do not know what a serving size looks like. At the very least have a look at the websites:

www.measureup.gov.au

www.eatright.org

www.webhost.sun.ac.za/nicus

www.5aday.co

www.eatforhealth.gov.au

Suggestions for healthy recipes:

Rocket Fuel on a Budget (Joanna Rushton)

I Quit Sugar (Sarah Wilson)

Healthy Every Day (Pete Evans)

The Whole Pantry (Belle Gibson)

Eat Real Food (David Gillespie)

Deliciously Ella (Ella Woodward)

Secrets of Feeding a Healthy Family (Ellyn Satter)

The Raw Food Kitchen (Amanda Brocket)

Everyday Super Food (Jamie Oliver)

Power Foods (Donna Hay)

The Naked Vegan (Maz Valcorza)

Some very basic suggestions:

Options for breakfast (alternatives to the regular toast or cereal)

- 285g of organic plain yoghurt, one piece of seasonal organic fruit (e.g. banana) and cinnamon
- or quinoa, amaranth and cocoa, and mixed berries
- or 2 scrambled eggs with mushrooms, tomato, spinach, capsicum peppers, and onion with herbs and spices
- or 1 cup of oatmeal with peaches, pears, apples

Options for morning snack and afternoon snack (about 3 hours after breakfast and lunch)

- seasonal fruit (e.g. apple)
- or a tablespoon of mixed nuts/seeds (e.g. Brazil nuts, almonds, hazelnuts, sesame seeds, pumpkin seeds, pepitas)
- or 1 hard boiled egg
- or a matchbox sized piece of cheese

Options for lunch: (alternatives to the regular sandwich)

- a salad made up of seasonal vegetables (e.g. lettuce, tomato, cucumber, sprouts, beetroot, ¼ avocado, celery, artichoke, spinach) drizzled with dressing made with 1tbsp of flax seed oil/Omega 3:6:9 oil, apple cider vinegar/balsamic vinegar, chives, spices, and herbs (e.g. cayenne pepper, garlic, parsley, fresh coriander)

- with 50g/palm sized piece of chicken
- or 1 serving/50 g (¼ tin) of tuna
- or mozzarella
- or feta cheese
- or seafood (shrimp, oysters, etc.)

Options for dinner: (alternatives to the regular rice and potatoes)

- Soup made up of blended vegetables (e.g. carrots, broccoli, turnips, parsnips, etc.) plus herbs and spices with meat
- Steamed or boiled vegetables (asparagus, pumpkin) with 80–120g cooked fish, meat, or seafood

The above is an example only. Add other foods, e.g. multigrain bread, brown rice, coffee, alcohol, and any treats (chocolates, cakes, biscuits) as desired—for specifics, please talk to a dietitian.

As a guide:

- Aim to have at least twenty different foods per day and don't have the same food two days in a row
- Aim to drink 2-3 litres of filtered water
- To calculate your daily calorie and nutrient requirements: Multiply your desired ideal body weight in kg by 2.2 to get pounds. Multiply this by 10 to obtain your goal daily calorie intake. For example, if you want to weigh 143 pounds (65kg), your daily goal calorie intake for weight loss would be 1,430 calories.

- **Protein requirement:** 40 percent of total intake needs to be from protein: multiply total calorie needs by 40 percent (e.g. 1430 x 40 = 572 calories). Then divide this by 4. Total protein needed: 143g
- **Carbohydrates requirement:** 30 percent needs to be from carbohydrates: multiply total calorie needs by 30 percent (1430 x 30 = 429 calories from carbs). Then divide this number by 4 (e.g. 540 ÷ 4 calories per gram = 107g of carbs daily).
- **Fat requirement:** 30 percent needs to be from fat: multiply daily caloric needs by 30 percent = 429 calories from fat. Now divide this number by 9 (e.g. 429 ÷ 9 calories = 48; thus 48g of fat is needed daily).
- **Fibre:** present in fruit, vegetables, oats, and wholewheat, the Dietitians Association of Australia recommends eating at least 25g of fibre per day. Researchers who reviewed 107 treatments on fibre concluded that high fibre intake is associated with lower body weight.[23]
- For more information on the pros and cons of specific diets, go to:
  - www.healthdirect.gov.au/diet-reviews
  - www.daa.asn.au
- Read all about whether there is such a thing as 'slimming foods' or 'fattening foods'; whether sugar is as evil as its made out to be; how we're being duped by the 'healthy' labels; whether to eat organic foods; how our hormones affect our weight; whether machines, supplements, and diet pills can accelerate slimming; how quitting smoking can actually help you lose weight in the *Hyp2Hip Slimming* book.

Chapter 16: **How the New Science in Exercise Can Boost Your Weight Loss**

'A dog is one of the few remaining reasons why some people can be persuaded to go for a walk.'
(O.A. Battista)

If you already exercise regularly, this chapter may provide you with some new insights and tricks to enhance your exercise experience to improve results even further. If, on the other hand, you struggle to get going with exercise, you probably have one or more of the following reasons for not exercising regularly or at all:

- You do not exercise because you 'don't have time'
- You shy away from a gym because you are too self-conscious when 'sweaty and smelly'; or fear being judged over your appearance, ability, and dress sense; or you afraid of looking silly in lycra
- You avoid exercise because you experience anxiety whilst exercising in public
- You ask 'what's the point?' or say 'I can't get motivated to do it'
- You are 'just too lazy' or don't like exercise
- You have a physical injury or pain that prevents you from exercising

If any of the above reasons apply to you, this chapter will inspire you to start on a new adventure that will give you the inspiration to continue on a regular exercise program that will work for you.

Is Exercise Really Necessary For Weight Loss and Maintenance?

Weight loss can occur without exercise. However, the facts on exercise and weight loss are as follows:

- According to the obesity management guidelines, the most effective approach to weight loss is to make behaviour changes that make it easier to eat fewer calories and become more active.[1]
- About 94 percent of people who lost weight and maintained it increased their physical activity, according to the National Weight Loss Registry (which is a database of 5,000 people who have lost an average of 70 pounds and kept it off for an average of 6 years). Of those 94 percent who exercise, about 90 percent exercise, on average, one hour per day with the most frequently reported form of activity as walking.[2]
- A Cochrane review of forty-three randomised controlled trials showed that exercise-only interventions can result in an average weight loss of 2kg compared with no treatment. Interventions that combine exercise and diet resulted in a greater reduction in weight than dietary interventions alone, with an average of 3kg loss. Increasing the intensity of the exercise increased weight loss by 1.5kg.[3]
- Diet alone can help you achieve and maintain your ideal weight. However, it is clear, without much exception, that a diet combined with exercise

will still provide you with the best result. As per a systematic review of six randomised controlled trials evaluating diet, or diet and exercise together, the results indicated an advantage to combined diet and exercise interventions which achieved a 20 percent greater sustained weight loss at one year compared to diet alone.[4]

- In a huge study of forty-five trials with 7,788 individuals investigated whether behavioural/lifestyle, pharmacological (e.g. Orlistat), food replacement/supplement, or alternative interventions were most effective. The researchers concluded that behavioural interventions focusing on both food intake and physical activity were the most effective.[5]
- Research reported in the *International Journal of Obesity* has confirmed you can increase your chances of weight loss with exercise: Italian researchers discovered that the probability of losing from 5–10 percent of initial weight increased by 20 percent for any 1,000 steps per day. The probability of losing more than 10 percent increased by over 30 percent. They also found metabolism (resting energy expenditure) increased by 100 calories per day even though they lost weight (usually metabolism reduces due to weight loss).[6]
- Finally, research has confirmed that the more exercise you do during a weight loss diet, the more likely it is that you will comply with a diet.[7]

You cannot undo bad eating with exercise but with a combination of diet and exercise, you are more likely to achieve and maintain your ideal weight/body.

THE Magic Trick to Perk up Your Exercise Motivation

If you've read the above reasons to exercise and don't feel motivated yet, here is the trick to get you excited about exercise: Canadian researchers have proven that visualising is a great way to get yourself motivated to exercise.[8] For some people—maybe for you—the thought about exercising is so much worse than actually doing it. Most people have great fun when they exercise, it's just about overcoming that inertia. Whether 'getting going' is the problem or whether it's fitting exercise in regularly, you can do a visualisation exercise to get through it. It takes only a few minutes: maybe 3 minutes. In fact, do it right now: close your eyes, visualise yourself intending to exercise, and having the usual excuses running through your head. Now, visualise yourself identifying that inertia and breaking through that, then getting into exercise gear and jumping up enthusiastically to exercise. The trick to making this exercise work for you is to visualise an exaggerated picture of your enthusiasm. If it doesn't work for you the first time, do it again.

Furthermore, as you are reading this, wondering how exercise is going to work for you, it's time to get excited about exercise: read all about the science behind the benefits of exercise, which type of exercise is best, for how long you should exercise to achieve results efficiently, when to exercise, how to stay safe during exercise, and how to stay motivated to exercise.

The Benefits of Exercise for Weight Management

Most of us have heard that exercise can break a weight loss plateau, but did you also know that exercise:

- ✓ Increases the capacity of muscle to oxidise fat[9]
- ✓ Prevents loss of muscle tissue (catabolism) during slimming regimes[10]
- ✓ Improves body fat distribution and reduces visceral fat deposits[11]
- ✓ Speeds up your metabolism (BMR) and energy expenditure (thermogenic response): the number of calories you burn through moderate exercise is about 15–30 percent above your resting metabolic rate[12]
- ✓ Increases levels of adiponectin, a hormone that helps to regulate metabolism and blood sugar levels. According to research published in *Obesity*, exercise can increase adiponectin levels by 260 percent in as little as one week[13]
- ✓ Decreases your appetite. Research published in the *Obesity* journal found that doing 5-minute bouts of exercise is an appetite suppressant: exercise that increases your heartbeat (e.g. power walking or climbing stairs) through the day made people feel 32 percent fuller in the afternoon[14]
- ✓ Exercise increases irisin, a hormone that not only reduces insulin resistance but also makes white fat behave more like brown fat, i.e. a calorie burner[15]
- ✓ Enhances the brain's executive function[16] (reasoning, planning ability), which means you will be better able to resist temptation

Bear in mind that while exercise does burn calories, exercise shouldn't be used to calculate how much you can eat. For example: you would have to run about 10km to burn off a chocolate muffin.[17] It's much better to calculate how much to exercise based on the other benefits of exercise.

Exercise has other benefits:

Apart from balancing your hormones and facilitating weight loss, other benefits of exercise include:

- ✓ Improved blood pressure, fasting glucose, and cholesterol[18]
- ✓ Reduced risk of cardiovascular disease, diabetes, some cancers, and mortality[19]
- ✓ Improved muscle and bone strength thus reducing your risk of falls[19]
- ✓ Reduced anxiety, depression, and sensitivity to stress[20]
- ✓ Improved immune system[21]
- ✓ Improved sleep[22]
- ✓ Improved self-esteem:[23] it provides you with a sense of achievement (e.g. by acquiring a new skill and having a sense of being 'good' at it)
- ✓ Reduced risk of dementia[24]
- ✓ Improved memory[25]
- ✓ Improved neuroplasticity and cognition[26]

How Will You Benefit From Exercise?

Having read above benefits from exercise, you may find that you benefit in many other ways too. For example, have you wondered about the opportunity to meet other people if you were to join running clubs, walking groups, rowing clubs, gyms? Which other non-physical benefits can you think of?

One objective way you can find out how you benefit from exercise—apart from change in muscle, water, fat, weight, and measurements—is to ask your GP to test your blood pressure, glucose, and cholesterol if you have not done so already. The other measure you may consider testing is Vo2 max, which is usually measured at gyms rather than in a doctor's office.

Resistance or Aerobic Exercise: Which Exercise is Best?

Researchers have found that intensive, high volume resistance training (but not aerobic training) prevents reductions in metabolism that usually accompany diet-induced weight loss.[27] At least one study has confirmed that adding strength training to your routine is best for fat loss as it increases muscle mass.[28] For example, one study reported in the journal *Clinical Obesity* investigated the effect of adding either aerobic training or resistance training to an educational weight management program on morbidly obese individuals. A total of 33 participants (aged 24 to 68 years with a BMI of 40kg) participated for 12 weeks. Both aerobic and resistance training proved to be effective in increasing fitness, self-efficacy, and interest/enjoyment. However, resistance training was more effective at decreasing waist measurements.[29]

In gyms I have attended, I've heard that personal trainers recommend that you do 30–40 minutes aerobic (e.g. running, cycling, swimming) sessions after weight session for maximum fat burning. I've also heard from various personal trainers that lifting lighter weights and doing 3 sets of 30 is as effective for muscle growth as lifting heavy weights for 8–12 reps. I have however, not found scientific evidence for this. To find out for yourself, go to an exercise physiotherapist.

Best Intensity of Exercise to Maximise Weight Loss

According to *The Journal of Strength and Conditioning Research*, the 'fat-burning' zone is exercising when your heart rate is between 105 and 134 beats per minute.[30] You can go on www.runnersweb.com

to calculate your target heart rate or observe the guideline about target heart rates according to the American Heart Association:[31]

Age	Target HR Zone 50–85%	Average Maximum Heart Rate 100%
20 years	100–170 beats per minute	200 beats per minute
30 years	95–162 beats per minute	190 beats per minute
35 years	93–157 beats per minute	185 beats per minute
40 years	90–153 beats per minute	180 beats per minute
45 years	88–149 beats per minute	175 beats per minute
50 years	85–145 beats per minute	170 beats per minute
55 years	83–140 beats per minute	165 beats per minute
60 years	80–136 beats per minute	160 beats per minute
65 years	78–132 beats per minute	155 beats per minute
70 years	75–128 beats per minute	150 beats per minute

If you don't have a heart rate monitor: you can find out if you're exercising too intensely by seeing if you're unable to talk while exercising.

Exercising too intensely can increase your chance of injury. Be sure to consult a GP or exercise physiologist, especially if you have health problems (e.g. pain, injuries, heart, or blood pressure problems).

Short and Sweet: The Best Way to Exercise

The conventional recommendation regarding exercise by the US Department of Health and Human Services and the Department of Health is 30 minutes of moderate-intensity physical activity five days per week.[32] This can be broken up into 10 minutes of incidental exercise, e.g. taking the stairs instead of the lifts, walking to the shop instead of driving, etc. However, short bouts of incidental exercise lasting 10–15 minutes are insufficient for preventing weight gain or weight loss or weight regain in most people.

According to the obesity management guidelines,[33] aerobic activity such as walking should be at least 150 minutes per week. To maintain lost weight or minimise weight regain long-term, greater amounts of physical activity (200-300 minutes per week) are recommended. The Canadian guidelines recommend 30 minutes of physical activity of moderate intensity per day, increasing to 60 minutes per day as part of an overall weight loss program, which should be both sustainable and tailored to the individual.[34] In Australia, the National Physical Activity Guidelines (2014) are as follows:[35]

- If you currently do no physical activity, start by doing some, and gradually build up to the recommended amount
- Be active on most days of the week; preferably all
- Each week engage in 2½–5 hours of moderate intensity physical activity (e.g. brisk walking, medium paced swimming or cycling) or 75–150 minutes (1¼–2½ hours) of vigorous intensity physical activity, or an equivalent combination of both moderate and vigorous activities

- Do muscle strengthening activities on at least two days each week

A study of 201 participants at the University of Pittsburgh Physical Activity and Weight Management Research Center concluded that for fat loss, 150 minutes per week of moderate intensity exercise is a good starting point, with the ideal duration per day (which is in line with the Institute of Medicine's recommendation) being 60 minutes.[36]

If the recommendation to exercise for an hour a day puts you off, you were probably attracted to the evidence in Dr Mosley's *Fast Exercise* book. Dr Mosley claims there's no need to exercise for long: in fact, he recommends workouts as short as four minutes! His argument is based on several studies that have proven that short bursts of exercise can have as much effect (or even better) than slower, longer workouts.

An example of a study on short duration exercise was done at the University of Wisconsin. Researchers concluded the 96 participants had improved aerobic fitness and muscle strength with only a 7 or 14 minute workout for 8 weeks.[37] Another study published in the *International Journal of Preventive Medicine* found that continuous exercise was less effective than intermittent exercise (short bursts of intense exercise followed by short rests periods).[38]

Several other studies have shown similar results. The emphasis though is that the workouts need to have short, intensive bursts. Although several investigators have experimented with different durations, there is a general consensus that high intensive intermittent exercise (HIIT) is much more effective than slow, steady, and long exercise. One study that investigated with a workout lasting 20 minutes with 8 seconds fast, 12 seconds rest was conducted at the University of New South Wales and the Garvan Institute. Compared to the participants who exercised for 40 minutes at a consistent pace, participants doing the HIIT lost more fat.[39]

Benefits of high intensity intermittent exercise (HIIT) compared to conventional exercise:

✓ More time efficient
✓ Reduces abdominal fat better[39]
✓ Improves insulin sensitivity faster[40]
✓ Builds muscle tone and improve fat loss faster[40]
✓ Suppresses appetite better[40]
✓ Speeds up your metabolism for up to 22 hours[41]

Fitness professionals have, of course, devised workouts based on the benefits of HIIT, e.g. 'Spartacus' workout and 'Insanity'. However, these HIIT-based workouts are much longer than the shorter workouts proposed by Dr Mosley.

Whereas most of the research confirms the superiority of HIIT, one study at the University of Sydney of 33 people found that a 12 week 24 minute HIIT workout is not as effective—at least to reduce abdominal fat—as traditional aerobic exercise (45 minute moderate pace exercise bike workout).[42] If you are now confused as to what to do, I would suggest you find what works for you. More importantly, find something you *enjoy*.

I personally enjoy doing the HIIT-based exercise DVD 'Insanity', every other day, alternated with 2 days of 40 laps in a 25m pool, one 30 minute run (continuous pace), and one 1 hour walk per week in addition to two daily walks (10–30 minutes) with my dog and cat (yes, the cat comes too!). You may be able to tell that I love exercise—hence, it is easy for me to do it. For a start, my cat insists on the morning walk and secondly, my dog insists on the evening walk. When I'm overseas, I go jogging. On my recent trip to Spain, I jogged every morning and got to know Spain in a different way that my fellow travellers did. I even got lost on two occasions, but thanks to my bit of knowledge in Spanish, I was able to find my way back to the hotel. I had a similar experience in Japan: I got lost jogging, but had a really nice time exploring Japan.

If you're currently not a fan of exercise and wonder how somebody can love it, continue to read so that you too can love it. You will love exercise when you start getting results. You will get results only when you're doing it and doing it right. Follow these instructions to get optimal results:

Optimal Time to Exercise

Most of us have heard that the best time to exercise is in the morning to boost metabolism and improve blood sugar levels. I have spoken to personal trainers who have recommended exercising after eating something (even if it's just a protein shake) as exercise on an empty stomach is not only detrimental to blood sugar levels, but also slows down metabolism and causes muscle (hence metabolism) waste. The facts on the timing of your exercise session are the following:

- Research at Kansas State University, found that more fat is burned in workouts prior to meals[43]
- According to a study by the University of Northumbria, working out before breakfast burns 20 percent more stored fat[44]
- Research published in the journal *Appetite* found that participants experienced a 30 percent greater

mood lift if they worked out in the morning compared to workouts in the evening[45]
- In regards to when and what to eat: research has confirmed that muscle growth was better when a protein-carbohydrate supplement was consumed immediately before exercise (compared to after)[46]

So, in deciding when to exercise: do it whenever it is that you're most likely to do it and can fit exercise into your routine. I personally find that I enjoy waking up early to exercise. I feel odd to shower without washing off sweat from a morning workout.

Staying Safe During Exercise

- Ensure you have the right clothing, equipment and footgear: To prevent injuries and maximise comfort and effectiveness
- Start slowly and set small, realistic goals: If you're not used to exercise, don't do too much too soon—ease into it or you'll be at risk of injury and burn out. It's best to ask your GP, an exercise physiologist, or a personal trainer what you can start out with. You can keep track of how fast/far you have run by using an app, e.g. www.runkeeper.com
- Go accompanied: If you are worried about safety (e.g. walking alone in the evening), go with a friend, colleague, neighbour, a dog, or take a self-defence class or know how to use your house keys for self-defence
- Stay safe: Avoid running or walking in the dark; if you end up in semi-darkness, ensure you run or walk close to streetlights where you can see where you're running and wear reflective clothing
- Always stretch after exercise: Do the right kind of stretching (and never bounce). Past president of

the Canadian Academy of Sport Medicine found that stretching before a workout actually led to reductions in muscle power. While stretching doesn't reduce your risk of injury if you're doing continuous exercise such as running/swimming, it's still recommended if you're doing a stop-start exercise (HIIT)[47]

- **Watch your form:** Don't do any exercise if you're not sure about whether you're doing it correctly. Form is very important to prevent injury. Consult an exercise professional, e.g. personal trainer or even better, an exercise physiologist
- **Watch out for pain:** It's normal to experience muscle soreness if you're not used to exercise. This will pass. However, if you feel joint pain, intense pain, or the pain persists beyond three days, see your GP
- **Check with your GP or exercise physiologist:** To see if there's any exercise you shouldn't be doing due to injuries or health conditions

22 Ways to Stay Motivated to Exercise

1. Just do 10 minutes

Starting can be the hardest part. This is the problem of inertia—getting going. Think about doing the housework ... then do it. Was it as bad as you thought it would be? The same thing can occur with exercise. Once you get going, you'll be fine. Never make the decision not to exercise while you're lying in bed. If you're going to make a decision about exercise in the morning, get up, go to the toilet, drink a glass of water, then decide to 'just do 10 minutes'. If you're not used to exercise, don't do an hour walk on your first day. Do 10 minutes the first day, then build up from there even if it's in increments of 5 minutes per day or week. I've seen too many people get burnt out or injured by doing too much too soon.

2. Do something you enjoy

If you didn't like the exercise you did, try something else until you find something you like. You can also find someone in your life who likes exercise. Find out how it is that he or she likes exercise and what exercise it is. Next time you meet a friend, arrange to meet for a walk rather than for coffee or lunch.

3. Exercise outdoors

Researchers at the University of Exeter Medical School found that exercising in a park, especially if it's near water, increases people's enjoyment of exercise.[48]

4. Jumble up what you do each day

To maintain interest in exercise and make your workouts more efficient at calorie burning, walk one day, do weight training the next, swim the next, etc.

5. If you prefer not to go alone

Take your dog, friend, neighbour, spouse, relative, colleague, or someone who'd like to join you. You could ask at least two of your colleagues to join a team and compete against another team of three. See if you have an employer is willing to provide a prize to the winning team. If you don't have a work team, get together with neighbours or friends to make up a competitive team. If you prefer online support, go to www.walkingwithattitude.com

6. Remind yourself of the benefits of exercise

Although exercise is only about 20 percent of weight loss, remember that you're not exercising only to lose weight. You're exercising for the other benefits too: e.g. stress relief, regulate your oestrogen, testosterone, insulin, etc.—see above benefits list.

7. Think about how much you'll regret not exercising

Research published in the *British Journal of Health Psychology* found that this is a very powerful motivator.[49]

8. Sign up for a charity walk or run

It's good for you and good for a charity.

9. Put exercise on the agenda of the day

Make it a habit: some people do it first thing in the morning so it's out of the way. Others prefer to do it after work to tune off from work. Exercise is best if you do it at the same time each day. For example, wake up at 6:15pm, exercise for 30 minutes then get ready for work. If you 'don't have time', do the quick exercises recommended by Dr Mosley or ensure that you change your day to fit in 30 minutes of exercise. There's nothing wrong with incidental exercise, e.g. using the stairs instead of the lifts, walking to shop, parking car furthest away, etc. I still think there's something wrong if you do not have 30 minutes to spare in your day to exercise. Apparently, even former Prime Minister Tony Abbott found time to exercise.

One of my patients, who came to me for a weight loss session, gave me the excuse 'no time'. He proceeded to tell me that he woke up at 5:30

a.m. because it took him 90 minutes to drive to work and 90 minutes to drive back home—no time in the morning, no time in the evening to exercise. We discussed ways around this, e.g. going for a walk at lunchtime. However, we finally concluded that his idea of living in a remote area (where he could relax) was actually causing him stress rather than the relaxation he sought living in the remote area. He was initially surprised, asking, 'So you're saying in order for me to lose weight, I need to move house?' On the surface, it does sound rather odd, but his stress levels from driving 180 minutes a day were higher than the relaxation he got from being at home for two days on the weekend. He agreed and put his house on the market. I heard back from him that he had sold his house (for a profit) and was now going to gym before work (only 30 minute drive to work). He also reported feeling much more relaxed.

I've had many people who will say they don't have time to exercise. When I ask them whether they can exercise in the morning, they will say, 'No, I have to leave the house at 7:30 a.m.' What do they do between waking up and leaving? Usually it involves hitting the snooze button for up to 30 minutes. In some cases it's because they care for everyone else except themselves. They wake up at 6 a.m., take care of the kids, and run their whole day accommodating others while having no 'me' time. If this sounds like you, make sure you make changes to take care of you. Lead by example.

10. Stop the excuses

I've heard people say, 'It's raining,' to which I reply, 'Do you have an umbrella?' In my case, rain is simply not an excuse because my dog, even my cat, demand a walk despite the rain. In summer, I actually like it if it rains when I go jogging as it washes off the sweat and keeps me cool. If you really don't like the idea of walking in the rain, make sure you have a backup plan for rainy or cold days, e.g. do a workout DVD at home in the comfort of your home.

11. Unlearn your old ritual

Bear in mind that if you haven't engaged in a particular activity (like jumping out of bed the minute the alarm goes off), it will be difficult to change that ritual. Fortunately, *any* activity you do can be unlearned. I use the word 'unlearned' because if you stay in bed after the alarm goes off, it's probably because you've trained yourself to do so for many weeks/months/years. The training initially involved you finding evidence for your behaviour, e.g. *I'm too tired, it's too cold, just a few more minutes to relax, it doesn't matter if I stay in bed longer, I won't enjoy it*, etc. The way you unlearn this behaviour is to find reasons for the opposite behaviour, i.e. jumping out of bed the minute you wake up. The first few days will involve you having to force yourself to do this together with evidence as to why it's good to do this, e.g. *it's not worth it to waste time in bed, it's cold anyway, I have to get up anyway*, etc. After a few days, you will notice that you will do this automatically. Some people find that giving themselves a penalty for getting out of bed late helps, e.g. having a cold shower. Others find that giving themselves a reward for getting out of bed helpful, e.g. buying a new pair of shoes.

I personally programmed myself to wake up without an alarm many years ago (I very rarely set it 'just in case'). I get out of bed within 5 minutes of waking unless I have not slept well (e.g. dogs barking, lightening, excitement about something, etc.). I walk my pets for 30 minutes, then do my formal exercise (about 38 minutes), and then only am I ready to start the day.

12. Keep going

If you have one day when you slip back into your old ritual, don't engage in 'all or nothing' thinking, i.e. *I didn't exercise today so I just can't do this*. Instead remind yourself, *it's just a little lapse* and get right back on track. Just do 10 push ups or sit ups while watching TV—something is better than nothing at all.

13. Reward yourself

Each time you overcome a hurdle, reward yourself, e.g. buy a new pair of shoes once you've gone to your first gym session.

14. Overcome morning fatigue

Most of my clients identify not having time to exercise due to feeling too tired to wake up earlier in the morning. Typically, morning fatigue can be due to a variety of factors including stress, dehydration, vitamin B deficiencies or iron deficiencies. If this applies to you, ensure you drink enough water, discipline yourself enough to go to bed (rather than sit up watching TV till late), and are nutritionally taking care of yourself.

15. Prioritise success over temporary embarrassment

Some people say to me they want to go to gym but 'feel too embarrassed about being so fat or sweaty' to even go to the gym. To this I say: What's more embarrassing: being fat or going to the gym to stop being fat? What's more important: your goal of managing your weight or your pride? In addition, for how long do you think you will feel embarrassed: 10 minutes, 30 minutes? How many other 'fatties' do you think you'll encounter? Do you really think you will be the only person in the gym who is not skinny? Will other people really be as bothered about you being fat or sweaty as much as you are? Even if they thought you look sweaty or fat—does it matter?

16. Get a reliable baby-sitter

I also have countless women who are mothers of kids of all ages who say they can't 'because of the baby' or 'because of the kids'. If your kids are the ones preventing you from taking care of yourself, how long do you think you can still care for them and be a good role model? If you have a baby, you can go for a walk with the stroller; or you can go to a gym that has day-care facilities; or you can drop them off at a trusted friend or relative. One patient told me that she doesn't have a friend or relative she can trust. This is a problem. If you don't have a friend you can trust, work on that as a goal.

17. Find an exercise that fits your budget

If it's an issue of money, make sure that you choose an exercise that fits your budget. Find out if your library has exercise DVDs, or go to garage sales to pick up exercise equipment (in working order), shop around for equipment online, or shop around for gym membership costs at various different gyms in your area (work or near home). Some gyms provide a two week free trial membership. Bear in mind that walking and running are FREE (apart from buying running shoes). If you don't like equipment or gym visits, try the fitness app body-weight workout 'PT in my pocket'.

18. Get feedback

Keeping track of calorie burn or steps with a pedometer may help you stay motivated. Tap dancing burns 400 calories an hour, polka 540, and swing dancing 300 per hour. Running burns 600 calories per hour. Be aware that certain cardio machine readouts are not accurate—according to the US Naval Health Research Centre.[50]

19. Exercise with your favourite music

Some gyms have treadmills and cycles with TV screens with regular TV channels as well as other interesting scenery on them, e.g. countryside of France.

20. Monitor your progress

Noting how you track between date A and date B can have a significant impact on your commitment. Different activity trackers are available: for example, the Trackfit (by Fortis) tracks steps, distance, as well as calories; the Pulse O2 (by Withings) checks heart rate in addition to steps. If you don't want a tracking device, a simple pedometer will keep track of how many steps you take (this can be stored on your mobile too). For example, a 30 minute walk is about 3,000 steps. Or you can note down how many push-ups or sit-ups, lunges, etc. you do at week 1, 2, 3, etc.

21. Wear something great

Wear clothing that not only fits but also makes you feel good. If you go to gym wearing an old, daggy, baggy tracksuit, you're unlikely to feel good. It need not be expensive.

22. 'Punish' yourself if you don't work out

If you are a parent, you will know how effective a punishment is to prevent recurrence of undesired behaviour, e.g. if you don't brush your teeth, I will remove your mobile phone for a day. You can give *yourself* a punishment if you don't exercise, e.g. shower in cold water if you don't exercise.

> Did you know that sitting is the 'new smoking'? According to research, sitting for many hours without getting up is bad for your health, increasing your risk of diabetes, heart disease, and early mortality even if you have physical activity in your day.[51] At work, you can remedy this by getting a standing workplace desk.[52] At home, notice how much time you spend sitting in front of the TV and see if you can do push-ups or other exercises while watching TV. If commuting, try standing on the train, or cycling or walking to work instead of sitting.

16. Exercise options

The most important thing about finding an exercise that will maximise your weight loss and management journey is to find an exercise you enjoy. If you don't enjoy the exercise you are doing, it can actually have the opposite effect.[53]

This week's exercise is to do one of the suggested physical activities—even if it's just *once*:

- Participate in a Zumba or SH-BAM class
- Get a trial membership at a women's gym (if you are a woman, of course) or a regular gym and ask for an orientation so that you know how to do the exercises
- Do a Qigong or Tai chi class or Tai Chi DVD (www.taichi18.com)
- Attend an Altitude Box, Circuit, Callanetics, aqua aerobics, Bootcamp, or aerobics class
- Go to a spinning class (Les Mills/cycling); the new trend of karaoke spin involves singing while cycling which apparently makes you control your breathing and helps you gauge whether you're going as intense and more too intensely than you need to be (you're not supposed to be able to sing easily while doing aerobic exercise—if you can, it means you need to go harder)
- Play a round of golf
- Do an exercise DVD (e.g. Psychocalisthenics) or Wii fit exercise. When looking for an exercise DVD, ensure the trainer has the right fitness professional credentials and start with ones that suit your fitness goals, e.g. Insanity, UFC Fit, and Jillian Michaels' Hard Body are for those more advanced compared to Brazil Butt Lift that may be better for starters
- Do aqua aerobics or swim laps
- Organise a personal trainer (www.fitness.edu.au) or go to www.meetyourpersonaltrainer.com.au to search for your location and training preferences
- Do a group personal training workout
- Use an exercise machine, e.g. elliptical trainer, bike, rowing machine, a rebounder, etc. and start out with 10 minutes (these can be bought at garage sales or fitness stores or on TV), working up to at least 30 minutes 5–7 days per week or alternate it with other exercises

- Take a walk with your dog, your partner, neighbour, friend, or alone (at least 10 minutes); or you can also join a walking group:
    - Contact the Heart Foundation at 1 300 362 787 or go to www.heartfoundation.org.au
    - To find a walking group in your area, your local city council may also offer walking groups
- Instead of meeting a friend/friends for coffee or lunch, meet for a walk along the beach, river, in the park, or around a nice neighbourhood or try water-walking ball or quidditch (a cross between rugby, tag, and dodgeball)
- Walk with weights or wear a weighted vest that's equivalent to 15 percent of your body weight (it will help you burn 12 percent more calories at a moderate pace of about 4 km per hour)
- If you have a dog, take a doggy boot camp class
- Go for a jog, or do a good deed and do exercise at the same time: join the Achilles Running Club which will pair you with people with physical disabilities; or go for a 15 minute jog at the nearest park or around a neighbourhood you like; or try backwards running, which is said to burn more calories and improve posture
- Try a Piloxing class (a combination of boxing, dance, and Pilates): www.piloxing.com
- Try dancing classes
- Do incidental exercise, i.e. walking to the shop down the road rather than driving, doing gardening, housework, taking the stairs instead of the lift, etc. Another form of incidental exercise is to work out your abdominal muscles by sitting up straight (rather than hunched over), walking 'tall' (with your head up straight and tummy tucked in), and standing up straight.

Glossary of Terms

Cochrane review: A summary of scientific research that synthesises results of the most recent methodologically sound studies.

Meta-analysis/meta-analytical review: A statistical technique for combining the findings from two or more randomised control trials to assess the clinical effectiveness of multiple interventions.

Morbid obesity: A BMI of over 40.

Obesity: An excess of body fat as expressed by BMI. BMI over 30 is considered obese.

Osmosis: This term is generally used to describe the process that causes a liquid (usually water) to pass through the wall of a living cell. However, it can also be used to describe an ability to learn and understand things gradually without much effort—'an unconscious assimilation'.

Successful weight loss: Maintaining a BMI below 18.5–24.9 for over one year. Health experts have also agreed that a loss of 5 percent of body weight can provide you with health benefits. For you, 'success' can mean whatever you want it to be.

Randomised controlled trial (RCT): A type of scientific study in which people are randomly allocated to either a treatment (or different types of treatment) and a control (no treatment/placebo) group. They typically involve large sample sizes (many people) rather than single or a few case studies, which helps the researcher generalise the results. For example, if a treatment is effective for 10 people, it doesn't necessarily mean the treatment is effective for you. But if the treatment is effective for 100 or even a 1,000 people, chances are it will be effective for you, as they are likely to have similarities to you. The RCT is considered the gold standard for a clinical trial as it reduces the chance that a result is due to chance.

Therapeutic alliance: Also known as 'rapport'; the relationship you have with your therapist.

What exactly is research?

You will notice that throughout this book, there many references to research that was conducted at various universities throughout the world. The reason for this is that *Weight Off Your Mind* is a slimming and binge eating elimination program that is based on science. Unlike other slimming books, *Weight Off Your Mind* is not based on a single research finding, nor is it based on something that a celebrity has said, it is not based on a weight loss strategy or pill or machine that works (supposedly for everyone). It has its foundation in evidence-based studies.

So what exactly is research? Research is usually done by specialists—usually at a university—to confirm a particular theory. Research that is considered to be reliable is published in scientific journals. The most reliable ones are then listed in a database called the Cochrane Database. They are said to be particularly valid if an article is 'peer reviewed' which means that other specialist peers look over it to ensure it's accurate. Some rogue researchers manipulate their statistics to support their hypotheses. This can be done in several ways. One way they can do this is to select their research participants from a particular area or population that are more likely to support their hypothesis. For example, if a researcher was to support the hypothesis that his diet product worked, he could just choose them from a gym (without mentioning that he did so). That's one of the reasons good studies will always provide exact information about where and how they recruited.

Researchers who ask leading questions or make participants give a socially desirable answer will also not provide valid results. For example, if a researcher was to ask participants if they washed their hands after going to the bathroom, most would answer yes even if they didn't. Being given financial incentives without revealing this in the research article is also considered invalid. For example, if Nescafe was to sponsor a study on the beneficial effect of coffee, would you believe the outcome? Unfortunately, many pharmaceutical companies have published results of medication without having it independently tested! Many diet supplements on the internet are being sold based on, 'studies that have shown x ingredient to be effective.'

Sadly, some researchers still delete, add, or outright alter their data to fit with their hypothesis. However, one of the worst things that I have seen—particularly in the hypnosis research—is basing a whole hypothesis on a study of too few people! In statistical terms, this is called power. Essentially, if you say that you did a certain treatment on only 10 people and it showed that is wasn't effective, it doesn't necessarily mean that the treatment isn't effective, it just means that you don't have enough people to base your theory on. I have also seen some interesting interpretations of studies; imagine reading an article that read: 'Slim Down With Rice'. The article supports its statement by saying that in China—which has rice as a staple diet—has an obesity rate less than 5 percent. Incidentally, if the headline read: 'Get Slim, Don't Speak English!' would you believe it based on the fact that in China less than 1 percent of the population speaks English? The correlation doesn't make sense and yet when a study was published that said that people who drink two or more cups of coffee per day had more sex, people believed that in order to have more sex, they need to drink more coffee!

Suggestions or claims made in *Weight Off Your Mind* are based on studies that have been conducted at universities and published in scientifically recognised journals. However, some have a high level of evidence and some only less. In some cases, I have outlined studies that have low level evidence, because I have further backed it up by case studies I have encountered in my practice. As noted in some chapters, e.g. Breathwork, Acupuncture, and TFT chapter, some treatments have very little research support and yet they work for some. Thus, while I usually back up my suggestions with solid pieces of evidence, you have to wonder why something works for some and not others and why the scientific community does not support the particular intervention.

Appendix I: **Tracking Your Progress**

Determine your goal weight

Research has found that maintainers are the ones who self-determine their weight.[1] This means that you have a greater chance of success if you are the one who determines your 'ideal' weight. You can look up your ideal weight in a chart, but this does not mean you have to get to that weight. Your happy weight is whatever you want it to be. In clinical practice, I have found that most of my patients choose a weight they have been before or they choose a weight that someone of their frame and age is. Set a weight range if you like and avoid striving for a weight goal that somebody else wants you to be.

Break down your ultimate goal into smaller short term goals

What may be helpful too is to set a realistic goal and break it down into smaller goals. A study of 385 people found that frequent goal setting focused specifically on diet or exercise was better than goal setting focused on weight loss per se.[2] In other words, if you focus on *strategies* to achieve your weight loss goal rather than just focusing on the goal weight, you are more likely to be successful. *Weight Off Your Mind* will guide you to identify and implement these strategies rather than what most other self-help books that just advise you to write down a goal weight and hope for the best. You may have heard of SMART goals: setting goals that are Specific, Measurable, Achievable, Realistic, and Time Limited, e.g. eat 5 servings of vegetables, 2 fruits a day; limit to 1,200 calories a day this week for 4 weeks to achieve goal 1 (65kg) by 01/10/2016; continue to increase exercise duration by 5 minutes each week for 4 weeks to achieve goal 2 by 04/11/2016. You will find out too that hypnosis too works best when you have specific strategies rather than just an end goal.

Weigh/measure yourself frequently

A study published in the *Journal of Health Psychology* found that weight monitoring may be useful for preventing weight gain.[3] The utility of weighing once weekly was also confirmed by the National Weight Loss Registry which found that 75 percent of maintainers weigh themselves at least once a week.[4] The fact that successful maintainers weigh themselves frequently is an indication that they use the scale as a tool that provides feedback to them.

How much weight do I need to lose each week?

If you are like many 'dieters' clinging onto outdated advice, you will be glad to know that *Weight Off Your Mind* may enlighten you with scientifically based facts that are likely to simplify your weight loss journey. For example, you may be familiar with the recommendation to lose weight gradually to prevent risking weight regain. This recommendation—to lose no more than ½ kg per week—was based on weight loss research that found this to be the case.[5] Although losing weight quickly leads to greater weight loss, some investigators have found that it is actually associated with more rapid weight regain than a gradual weight loss.[6]

However, a study at the University of Florida of 298 women found that those who lost weight at a fast rate (more than 1.5 lbs/~0.6kg per week) during the first 4 weeks achieved greater weight reductions at 6 months than those who lost at slower rates (0.5 lbs or less). At 18 months follow up, those who had lost weight rapidly also maintained a significantly greater weight loss than those who had lost more gradually.[7]

In addition, researchers at the University of Melbourne investigated the effects of rapid versus gradual weight loss on 204 obese participants.[8] Although the results showed that both rapid and gradual weight loss group participants had the same rate of success at 144 weeks follow up (24 percent were maintaining), the participants who followed the rapid weight loss plan had greater success in losing weight: 83 percent of the rapid weight loss group (on 800 calories in 12 weeks) lost 1.5kg a week. This is compared to only 50 percent of the slower weight loss group (losing 0.5 kg a week for 36 weeks) who achieved their goal weight. The researchers found an additional benefit in the group on the quick weight loss: the low calorie diet tended to suppress appetite!

Thus, the research indicates that losing weight rapidly may not only improve your success at actually achieving weight loss (and suppressing your appetite), it may also increase your chance of maintaining it. In my clinical practice, I have found that both rapid and gradual weight loss works. However, I have definitely found that those who lose weight rapidly are those who have finally changed their old eating behaviours and thus have the weight almost literally 'dropping off'. Of course, I have seen with my patients that those over 100 kg lost more weight per week than those who needed to lose only about 10–25 kg and weight loss is always greater in the first 2–3 weeks. Do whatever works for you. Cautionary note: always check with your medical professional to ensure that the weight loss strategy you are commencing is healthy and safe and is focused on fat loss, not muscle (and mostly water) loss. Remember that looking at your scale for 'weight' loss may not be the best strategy anyway (see further details on the section below about how to measure fat/weight loss).

If you find the idea of weighing yourself scary, you are like many of the patients who have come to me to address weight management problems. Rest assured: I will provide you with tools to overcome this 'phobia' about scales. It is, however, important to know that overcoming this 'scale phobia' is important. I see it as similar to an alcoholic not wanting to listen to feedback from the Dr about liver function test results. Just like a liver function test that provides feedback about the damage done by excessive alcohol consumption, the scale too can provide you with information about what has been going on for you. It does tend to break through that safety net called denial. I know weighing yourself again—especially if it has been a long time and you believe you have gained—may not be easy.

If you do have a fear of stepping onto the scale, be sure to use the psychological methods—you will then be able to notice, either suddenly or gradually, that you are becoming friends with your scale. If you are currently fearful of the scale or just have a bit of trepidation: the time to start weighing yourself regularly is when you are ready. If you are not ready today, do it when you are. Here are some tips about weighing yourself:

- Weighing yourself on a digital scale is preferable to a mechanical scale as the former also measures body fat, muscle mass, and water mass which provides you with more accurate feedback as to whether the weight that you are losing is fat or just water; it can also provide you with an explanation for weight gain which may in fact be muscle, not fat. For example, you may have lost 1kg of fat but gained 1kg of muscle but your scale is telling your mechanical scale is telling you that you haven't changed!
- You may notice weight increases due to water retention caused by high sodium (salt) intake, air pressure from flying for more than 4 hours, or premenstrual weight, which can be as much as 2kg of water.
- Your body mass index (BMI) is not the best way to measure your current status. However, if you would like to calculate your BMI, you can do so by doing this calculation: weight (in pounds) x 700 divided by your height (in inches) squared (or try websites to help you calculate, e.g. www.scientificpsychic.com)
- Weigh yourself first thing in the morning without clothes and prior to eating and drinking anything but after using the toilet
- Avoid weighing yourself more than once a week
- Colonic hydrotherapy session may, apparently, make you 'lose' 1kg or more of faecal matter from your bowels

- In regards to how much body fat is healthy, depending on which charts you look up, a healthy body fat range for women is as low as 8 percent and as high as 31 percent, depending on age (the older, the more fat). However, most charts will say a healthy range is 18–31 percent. For men, also depending on age, it ranges from 5–20 percent fat. The gold standard nowadays of weight measurement is the DXA (dual-energy X-ray absorptiometry) scan, which can be performed by radiologists. Otherwise a regular scale or a digital scale that measures fat percentage can be used.
  - Even better than BMI or a simple weight are measurements. Take a tape measure to measure your arm, bust/chest, waist, hip, and thigh. Ensure that you note a spot on each place so that you measure the same place each time (e.g. along a freckle). You may find that you do not lose weight one week but lose centimetres. Go to www.australia.gov. au/ MeasureUp or look up the The Ashwell Shape Chart. According to www.shapeup.gov.au, a woman's waist measurement should be below 80cm and a man's below 94cm.
  - On the tracking sheet, fill in your current weight and measurements

How can I prevent weight regain?

Weight Off Your Mind is focused on eliminating the root cause of your binge eating/overeating/weight problems. Just as pulling out a weed at the root prevents regrowth, removing the cause of your problem with the hypnosis and other methods outlined in *Weight Off Your Mind* will eliminate the symptoms. Researchers who have investigated physiological reasons for weight regain have found that weight maintenance may be difficult as the metabolism does not reset once a lower weight is achieved and may even strengthen with time during weight maintenance.[9] Indeed, most people find that after dieting, they relapse into old eating patterns and regain weight due to increased appetite, hunger, and cravings.[10] The 'broken set point' theory explains how, with reduced calorie intake, dieters go into a 'famine reaction'. Part of your brain called the 'hypothalamus' responds by: increasing hunger and cravings (double in men), increasing lethargy, slowing down metabolism, decreasing thyroid function, and increasing cortisol (the stress hormone).

In most people, the Famine Reaction works in reverse too i.e., when weight is regained past set point, hunger and appetite and hence weight decrease until the set point weight is reached. This mechanism seems to be disturbed in some people—hence, the name 'broken set point'.[11] In other words, you have to work even harder to maintain the lower weight.[12]

It's also been proposed that success is far more likely for those who need to lose only 5–15 pounds (~2.5–7kg) because the adjustment in physiological set point is so modest.[13] However, this has not been supported so much in the scientific literature. Many case studies have provided evidence that achieving an ideal/happy body/weight can be achieved even by people who need to lose vast amounts of weight.

However, remember that I noted that the evidence for the broken set point theory was investigated by researchers who were investigating the *physical reasons* that weight maintenance could be experienced as difficult. Rest assured: your weight loss story is so much more than your physiology! Again, a reminder that this book is about using your mind power to conquer your weight management problem.

Tracking Sheet

DATE	WEIGHT	FAT	MUSCLE	WATER

ARMS	WAIST	HIPS	THIGHS

Appendix 2: **Monitor Your Behaviours**

Researchers have identified that maintainers are successful at maintaining because they monitor their eating behaviours.[1] You may not notice how much you are eating or even what you are eating when you eat mindlessly, e.g. while cooking, while watching TV, while sitting talking to friend. Monitoring your food intake, even just for a day, can help you 'catch' yourself become more alert to your intake. Self-monitoring can also be helpful if you don't know why you are overweight—you may think you don't eat much but when you monitor your food intake, it should help you identify where all the calories are coming from.

You can monitor your eating through a simple self-monitoring sheet in which you note what you eat, even for 1–3 days only. You can download a self-monitoring sheet at www.cci.health.wa.gov.au, then click on Resources (Consumers), then Overcoming Disordered Eating (Part A) Module 4: Self-Monitoring. Alternatively, if you prefer a hard copy, start an eating journal in which you write down what you ate when, whether you binged, and what thoughts and feelings you had with the meal.

Monitoring your behaviours and weight is also helpful to help you stay on track

According to research at the National Weight Control Registry, maintainers tend to stay within 2kg of their weight. Those who had not relapsed or gained after 1 year were the ones who kept it off long term.[2] In other words, if you gain 1–2 kg and lose track, you are on a slippery slope back to your baseline weight. Maintainers are the ones who catch lapses and change their ways immediately rather than going with the 'what the hell' attitude. They get back on track immediately. If you have ever regained weight due to going from a little lapse to a full blown relapse, you will find the strategies in *Weight Off Your Mind* will assist you in preventing this cycle.

Appendix 3: **Alcohol and Your Weight**

In my clinical experience with people who have attended sessions with me for weight problems, previous failures to maintain weight are sometimes due to these two factors: stressful events and being exposed to a favourite food, especially when also drinking alcohol. Stress and alcohol in combination then makes them slip back into old behaviours. Even eating one little bit of chocolate while tipsy leads to bingeing. This is similar to what I have seen with my drug addicts—'one is too many and a thousand is never enough'.

If alcohol was responsible for your past weight management failure/relapse, evaluate if alcohol is a major or even the main problem. Was alcohol used as a problem solver? Was it just an excuse? Did you let down that guard that you needed to stay on track? Maybe you just need to avoid having your favourite food around when you are drinking alcohol?

If you know for certain that alcohol is not the main problem, you may nevertheless know that alcohol can interfere with rational decision making. Researchers at the University of Alabama at Birmingham found that some people have more frequent impulsive eating behaviours the more alcohol is consumed in one sitting.[1] A study by the Department of Neuroscience at Uppsala University in Sweden discovered—by reviewing three meta-analyses—that alcohol affects your thinking and therefore impairs your ability to control your food intake.[2]

If you drink alcohol occasionally, your weight and appetite should not be affected a great deal. It may be worth keeping in mind though that alcohol is relatively high in calories content: a 200ml serving/1 glass of wine = 150 calories; a 300 ml serving of beer = 96 cal.[3] But drinking 400 ml (2 glasses) of wine is the equivalent of a light meal in terms of calories but is neither filling nor does it have nutritional value. Whereas you may believe that wine can be good for you because of its 'heart benefitting resveratrol', you are better off eating grapes as they contain the beneficial resveratrol too without damaging your brain like alcohol does.

Alcohol can cause a variety of health problems including liver damage if consumed in excess. However, a sedentary lifestyle and a diet that is high in calories, sugar, and fat intake can also cause liver damage or non-alcoholic fatty liver disease (NAFLD). The higher your body mass index (BMI), the greater the liver damage. Although the early stages of a fatty liver are symptomless, in the late stages, symptoms include liver failure, swelling of the legs (oedema), accumulation of fluid in the abdomen, bleeding from veins in the oesophagus, and mental confusion. Advanced stages also increases the risk of developing liver cancer.[4]

If you drink alcohol occasionally and/or have an unhealthy diet, ask your GP to do a Liver Function Test (LFT) to provide you with biofeedback on how your drinking and unhealthy eating is affecting your liver and the rest of your body. You do not have to stop drinking alcohol to succeed at slimming (unless you have an alcohol use disorder)

If you drink more than two standard alcoholic drinks 5 days a week and feel that you can't stop drinking, discuss it with your GP or another health practitioner. Your chance of success with weight management is significantly less if you currently have a drinking problem. However, help is available—start by asking for appropriate help. If you're in control of your drinking but struggle to control your food intake when you're drinking, make a decision: either drink or eat. Take the AUDIT below to check out if drinking is a problem. Keep in mind that even if your liver does not show up as a problem, drinking excessively (more than 2 standards drinks 5 days per week) especially for extended periods, can not only decrease your chances of losing weight, it can also have other very negative and devastating physical and mental health effects.

If you drink excessively and cannot stop on your own, there are several options for treatment, depending on your level of dependence: ask your GP for Antabuse as well as Campral or Revia; in addition, ask your GP to refer you to a psychologist or detoxification and/or rehabilitation for addiction treatment or outpatient psychological treatment; attend at least two Alcoholics Anonymous (A.A.) meetings.

How to succeed at slimming

Do not continue the *Weight Off Your Mind* program if you drink excessively and cannot stop or limit it to two standard drinks 5 days per week. If you drink alcohol excessively, ask your GP for help. **Get treatment for your alcohol addiction prior to continuing Weight Off Your Mind.**

Take the AUDIT to see if your drinking is risky:

AUDIT[3]	0	1	2	3	4
1. How often do you have a drink containing alcohol?	Never	Monthly or less	2–4 times a month	2–3 times a week	4 or more times a week
2. How many alcoholic drinks do you have on a typical day when you are drinking?	1 or 2	3 or 4	5 or 6	7–9	10 or more
3. How often do you have 6 or more drinks on one occasion?	Never	Less than monthly	Monthly	Weekly	Daily or almost daily
4. How often during the past year have you found that you drank more or for a longer time than you intended?	Never	Less than monthly	Monthly	Weekly	Daily or almost daily
5. How often during the past year have you failed to do what was normally expected of you because of your drinking?	Never	Less than monthly	Monthly	Weekly	Daily or almost daily
6. How often during the past year have you had a drink in the morning to get yourself going after a heavy drinking session?	Never	Less than monthly	Monthly	Weekly	Daily or almost daily

AUDIT[3]	0	1	2	3	4
7. How often during the past year have you felt guilty or remorseful after drinking?	Never	Less than monthly	Monthly	Weekly	Daily or almost daily
8. How often during the past year have you been unable to remember what happened the night before because of your drinking?	Never	Less than monthly	Monthly	Weekly	Daily or almost daily
9. Have you or anyone else been injured as a result of your drinking?	No		Yes, but not in the past year		Yes, during the past year
10. Has a relative, friend, doctor, or health care worker been concerned about your drinking or suggested that you cut down?	No		Yes, but not in the past year		Yes, during the past year

If your score is 8 or above, your drinking is considered to be at 'risky' levels.

Appendix 4: **Night Eating Syndrome, Bulimia Nervosa, and Sleep-Related Eating Disorder**

Weight Off Your Mind is targeted at people who have weight problems and/or struggle with overeating, binge eating, or have actual Binge Eating Disorder. Although Bulimia Nervosa and Night Eating Syndrome have some similarities, it is beyond the scope of this book. If you are not sure, go through the following checklists then seek treatment from a qualified psychologist. You can find a psychologist at www.psychology.org.au. The checklists are not diagnostic tests. They are a guideline only, based on the Diagnostic and Statistical Manual (DSM-5). Only a qualified mental health care professional (psychologist, psychiatrist) can diagnose. If you do not meet any of these criteria, but are still concerned about your weight/shape or body, seek help from a qualified psychologist.

Night Eating Syndrome (NES)[1]	Check yes if this occurred in the past 3 months
At least 3 times per week, you eat high calorie snacks/foods (at least one third of your daily calories) after the last daily meal, i.e. you wake up from sleep to eat	
Your appetite is poor in the morning	
You eat at least 50 percent of calories in the evening	

Treatment for night eating disorder (NES) has not been evaluated adequately. So far, the medication Sertraline has been trialed.[2] Cognitive Behavioural Therapy (CBT)[3] and relaxation training[4] are the non-pharmacological options.

Bulimia Nervosa[5]	Check if yes
You binge eat at least twice weekly for 3 months (binge eating is defined as eating a large amount of food and having a sense of loss of control over eating)	
You regularly use laxative, vomiting, diuretics, fasting, exercise, or other means to compensate for eating too much	
Your self-esteem is dependent on your body/shape/weight	

The treatment options for bulimia nervosa (BN) include anti-depressants[6], cognitive behavioural therapy (CBT)[7], and mindfulness-based therapies.[8] Other options may be available. Although treatment options mentioned in *Weight Off Your Mind* may be suitable for NES or BN, it is best to consult a clinician specialised in these disorders to clarify.

Sleep-related eating disorder (SRED) is characterised by recurrent episodes of waking up to eat. Foods consumed may either be high calorie foods, even toxic or inedible foods. Most people do not remember anything at all or only have vague memory of eating. Thus, they do not know why they gain weight. Some people also engage in sleepwalking, have restless legs syndrome, obstructive sleep apnoea syndrome, or use sleeping tablets. Treatment includes anti-depressants (SSRIs, e.g. 20–30mg per day); Topiramate (100–300mg); or clonazepam (0.5–2.0mg). Those who have restless legs may benefit from Pramipexole, while sleepwalking-related SRED benefits from Clonazepam.[9]

Appendix 5: **Feedback Form**

I would love to hear from you! Once you complete *Weight Off Your Mind* let me know how much weight you've lost, for how long you've maintained it, quit binge eating, had other pleasant side-effects, or any other comment. I would really appreciate your feedback to assist me in tracking what works. Please complete this form and return it to: doctor-katierichard@hotmail.com.

1. Did you lose weight because of Weight Off Your Mind?

Please circle the response that applies to you:

1. Yes, my initial weight was _____ kg and is now ____ kg (I lost _____kg).
2. No, I didn't lose weight/yes, I lost _____ kg but __

____

____

____

____

2. Did you stop binge eating? Have you been able to moderate your food intake?

Please circle the response that applies to you:

Yes No

Which part of *Weight Off Your Mind* was the most effective for you?

____

____

____

____

3. Have there been any improvements in mood, stress or anxiety? Circle which one(s):

Please circle the response that applies to you:

Mood

0---------- 1 ----------2---------------------- 4 ----------5
Not at all Some improvement A great deal

Stress

0---------- 1 ----------2---------- 3---------- 4 ----------5
Not at all Some improvement A great deal

Anxiety

0----------------------2---------- 3---------- 4 ----------5
Not at all Some improvement A great deal

4. Have there been any improvements in your physical health?

Yes (describe): ______________________________

____

No

5. Has your attitude toward food changed since *Weight Off Your Mind?*

0---------- 1 ----------2---------- 3---------- 4 ----------5
Not at all Some improvement A great deal

6. Do you feel better about your body and/or yourself?

0----------- 1 -----------2----------- 3----------- 4 -----------5
Not at all Some improvement A great deal

Any other comments, suggestions, complaints, compliments?

____

____

____

____

Sources

Introduction

1. Cochrane, A. (2014). Eating Disorder and Obesity Conference in Queensland in May. Multicomponent programs
2. Franz, M.J. and Van Womer J.J., et al. (2007). Weight-Loss Outcomes: Systematic Review and Meta-Analysis of Weight-Loss Clinical Trials with a Minimum 1-Year Follow-Up. *Journal of the American Dietetics Association,* 7 (10): 1755-1767.
3. Strychar, I., Lavoie, M.-E., Messier, L. et al. (2009). Anthropometric, metabolic, psychosocial, and dietary characteristics of overweight/obese post-menopausal women with a history of weight cycling: a MONET (Montreal Ottawa New Emerging Team) study. *Journal of the American Dietetic Association*, 109: 718–724.
4. Cochrane, G. (2008). Role for a sense of self-worth in weight-loss treatments: Helping patients develop self-efficacy. *Canadian Family Physician*, 54(4), 543-547.
5. Hemmingsson, E., Johansson, K. & Reynisdottir, S.(2014). Effects of childhood abuse on adult obesity: a systematic review and meta-analysis. *Obesity Reviews.* DOI: 10.1111/obr.12216.
6. Elfhag, K. and Rössner, S. (2005). Who succeeds in maintaining weight loss? A conceptual review of factors associated with weight loss maintenance and weight regain. *Obesity Reviews*, 6, (1) 67–85.

7. Wing, R.R. and Phelan, S. (2005). Long-term weight loss maintenance. *American Journal of Clinical Nutrition*, 82, 1222S-225S.
8. Elfhag, K. and Rössner, S. (2005). Who succeeds in maintaining weight loss? A conceptual review of factors associated with weight loss maintenance and weight regain. *Obesity Reviews*, 6, (1) 67–85.
9. Wing, R.R. and Hill, J.O. (2001) Successful weight loss maintenance. *Annual Review of Nutrition*, 21: 323–341.
10. Befort, C.A.,Stewart, E.E., Smith, B.K., Gibson, C.A., Sullivan, D.K., Donnelly, J.E.(2008). Weight maintenance, behaviors and barriers among previous participants of a university-based weight control program. *International Journal of Obesity*, 32,519–526; doi:10.1038/sj.ijo.0803769
11. Klem, M.L., Wing, R.R.,Lang, W., McGuire, M.T. and Hill, J.O. (2000). Does Weight Loss Maintenance Become Easier Over Time? *Obesity Research*, 8:438–444.
12. Jeffery, R. W., Epstein, LH., Wilson, G. T, Drewnowski, A., Stunkard, A. J.; Wing, R.R. (2000). Long-term maintenance of weight loss: Current status. *Health Psychology*, 19(1), Suppl), 5-16. http://dx.doi.org/10.1037/0278-6133.19.Suppl1.5
13. Wing, R.R. and Phelan, S. (2005). Long-term weight loss maintenance. *American Journal of Clinical Nutrition*, 82, 1 222S-225S.
14. Douketis, J. D., Macie, C., Thabane, L., & Williamson, D. F. (2005). Systematic review of long-term weight loss studies in obese adults: clinical significance and applicability to clinical practice. *International Journal of Obesity*, 29(10), 1153-1167.
15. The NHLBI and NAASO (2013). The Practical Guide: Identification, Evaluation, and Treatment of Overweight and Obesity in Adults. Pub ID: 00-4084.

Chapter 1: Dr to the Rescue

1. Canaris, G.J, Manowitz, N.R, Mayor, G. & Ridgway, E.C. (2000). The Colorado thyroid disease prevalence study. *Archives of Internal Medicine*, 28: 526–342.
2. Rodin, J., Wack, J., Ferrannini, E., DeFronzo, R.A.(1985). Effect of insulin and glucose on feeding behavior. *Metabolism*. 34(9), 826-31.
3. The Australian Diabetes, Obesity and Lifestyle study (AusDiab) 2000.
4. Abstracts of the 19th European Congress on Obesity (ECO2012). Lyon, France. May 9-12, 2012. *Obesity Facts*, 5 Suppl 1:1-280. doi: 10.1159/000178121.
5. Salehpour, A., Farhad Hosseinpanah, F., Shidfar, F., Vafa, M., Razaghi, M., Dehghani, S., Hoshiarrad, A. and Gohar. M. (2012). A 12-week double-blind randomized clinical trial of vitamin D3 supplementation on body fat mass in healthy overweight and obese women. *Nutrition Journal*, 11: 78, 1-8.
6. Ortega, R. M., Aparicio, A., Rodríguez-Rodríguez, E., Bermejo, L. M., Perea, J. M., López-Sobaler, A.,M., . . . Andrés, P. (2008). Preliminary data about the influence of vitamin D status on the loss of body fat in young overweight/obese women following two types of hypocaloric diet. The *British Journal of Nutrition*, 100(2), 269-72.
7. Salehpour, A., Farhad Hosseinpanah, F., Shidfar, F., Vafa, M., Razaghi, M., Dehghani, S., Hoshiarrad, A. and Gohar. M. (2012). A 12-week double-blind randomized clinical trial of vitamin D3 supplementation on body fat mass in healthy overweight and obese women. *Nutrition Journal*, 11: 78, 1-8.
8. Slusher, A. L., Mcallister, M. J., & Huang, C. (2015). A therapeutic role for vitamin D on obesity-associated inflammation and weight-loss intervention. *Inflammation Research*, 64(8), 565-575. doi:http://dx.doi.org/10.1007/ s00011-015-0847-4.

9. Heaney, R.P., K., Davies, M. & Barger-Lux J.(2002). Calcium and Weight: Clinical Studies. *Journal of the American College of Nutrition*, 21(2), 152S-155S.
10. Gallo, M.F., Lopez, L.M., Grimes, D.A, Carayon, F, Schulz, K.F., Helmerhorst, F.M. 2014). Combination contraceptives: effects on weight (Review). The Cochrane Database of Systematic Reviews, 1. Art. No.: CD003987. DOI: 10.1002/14651858.CD003987. pub5.
11. Bak, M., Fransen, A., Janssen, J., Os, J. and van Drukker, M. (2014). Almost all Anti-psychotics result in weight gain: A Meta-Analysis. PLoS ONE 9(4): e94112. doi:10.1371/journal.pone.0094112.

Chapter 2: Self-Efficacy: Know That You Can

1. Shin, H., Shin, J., Liu, P., Dutton, G. R., Abood, D. A., & Ilich, J. Z. (2011). Self-efficacy improves weight loss in overweight/obese postmenopausal women during a 6-month weight loss intervention. *Nutrition Research*, 31(11), 822-828.doi:http://dx.doi.org/10.1016/j.nutres.2011.09.022
2. Karoly, P. Anderson, C. Wheeler, Snyder, C. R. (Ed); Ingram, Rick E. (Ed), (2000). The long and short of psychological change: Toward a goal-centered understanding of treatment and durability and adaptive success. *Handbook of psychological change: Psychotherapy processes & practices for the 21st century*. (pp. 154-176). Hoboken, NJ, US: John Wiley & Sons Inc, xvi, 768 pp.
3. Snyder, C. R. (2002). Hope theory: Rainbows in the mind. *Psychological Inquiry*, 13, 249-275.
4. Latner, J. D., & Ciao, A. C. (2014). Weight-loss history as a predictor of obesity treatment outcome: Prospective, long-term results from behavioral, group self-help treatment. *Journal of Health Psychology*, 19(2), 253-261. doi:http://dx.doi.org/10.1177/1359105312468191

5. Carpenter, M. J., Jardin, B. F., Burris, J. L., Mathew, A. R., Schnoll, R. A., Rigotti, N. A., & Cummings, K. M. (2013). Clinical strategies to enhance the efficacy of nicotine replacement therapy for smoking cessation: A review of the literature. *Drugs*, 73(5), 407-26.
6. Wetter, D.W., Fiore, M. C., Gritz, E. R., Lando, H. A., Stitzer, M. L., Hasselblad, V., & Baker, T.B. (1998). The agency for health care policy and research smoking cessation clinical practice guideline: findings and implications for psychologists. *The American Psychologist*, 53(6), 657-669.
7. Armitage, C. J., Wright, C. L., Parfitt, G., Pegington, M., Donnelly, L. S., & Harvie, M. N. (2014). Self-efficacy for temptations is a better predictor of weight loss than motivation and global self-efficacy: Evidence from two prospective studies among overweight/ obese women at high risk of breast cancer. *Patient Education and Counseling*, 95(2), 254-258. doi: http:// dx. doi.org/10. 1016/j.pec.2014.01.015
8. Harris, W.S., Gowda, M., Kolb, J.W., Strychacz, C.P., Vacek, J.L., Jones, P.G., Forker, A., O'Keefe, J.H., McCallister B.D.(1999). A Randomized, Controlled Trial of the Effects of Remote, Intercessory Prayer on Outcomes in Patients Admitted to the Coronary Care Unit. *Archives of Intern Med.* 159(19):2273-2278. doi:10.1001/ archinte. 159.19.2273.
9. Damisch, L., Stoberock, B., & Mussweiler, T. (2010). Keep your fingers crossed! How superstition improves performance. *Psychological Science*, 21 (7), 1014-1020. DOI: 10.1177/0956797610372631

Chapter 3: Feeding Your Self-Esteem, Not Your Stomach

1. De Zwaan, M., Mitchell, J.E., Seim, H.C., Specker, S.M., Pyle, R.L., Raymond, N.C. & Crosby, R.B. (1994). Eating related and general psychopathology in obese females with binge eating disorder. *International Journal of Eating Disorders*, 15,43-52.

2. Polivy, J. & Herman, C.P. (1985). Dieting and binging: A causal analysis. *American Psychologist*, 40,193-201.
3. Mcallister, R. and Caltabiano, M.L. (1994). self-esteem, body-image and weight in noneating-disordered women. *Psychological Reports*, 75, 9, 1339-1343. doi: 10.2466/pr0.1994.75.3.1339.
4. Kelly, A.C. Vimalakanthan, K. and Carter, J.C.(2014). Understanding the roles of self-esteem, self-compassion, and fear of self-compassion in eating disorder pathology: An examination of female students and eating disorder patients. *Eating Behaviors*, 15 (3), 388–391
5. Kelly, A.C. & Carter, J.C. (2012). Why self-critical patients present with more severe eating disorder pathology: The mediating role of shame. *British Journal of Clinical Psychology*, 52, 2, 148–161. DOI:10.1111/bjc.12006
6. Hrabosky, J. I., Masheb, R.M., White, M. A; Grilo, C. M. (2007). Overvaluation of Shape and Weight in Binge Eating Disorder. *Journal of Consulting and Clinical Psychology*, 75(1), 175.

Chapter 4: Slimming by Social Osmosis

1. Kayman, S., Bruvold, W. and Stern, J.S.(1990). Maintenance and relapse after weight loss in women: behavioral aspects. Am J Clin Nutrition, 52,(5), 800-807 .
2. Elfhag K, Rossner S.2005). Who succeeds in maintaining weight loss? A conceptual review of factors associated with weight loss maintenance and weight regain.Obesity Rcview, 6:67– 85.
3. Williamson, D.A. & Stewart, T.M. (2005). Behavior and lifestyle: approaches to treatment of obesity. Europe PubMed Central. 157 Spec No 1:S50-5.
4. Greaves, C. J., Sheppard, K. E., Abraham, C., Hardeman, W., Roden, M., Evans, P. H., & Schwarz, P. (2011). Systematic review of reviews of intervention

components associated with increased effectiveness in dietary and physical activity interventions. *BMC Public Health*, 11, 119. doi:http://dx.doi.org/10.1186/1471-2458-11-119.

5. Garssen, B. (2004) Psychological factors and cancer development: evidence after 30 years of research. *Clin Psychol Rev*, 24:315–338.
6. Christakis, N.A., and Fowler, J.H. (2007). The Spread of Obesity in a Large Social Network over 32 Years. *New Engl J Med,* 357:370-379DOI: 10.1056/NEJMsa066082.
7. Hayes, S. C., Rosenfarb, I., Wulfert, E., Munt, E. D., Korn, Z., & Zettle, R. D. (1985). Self-reinforcement effects: An artifact of social standard setting? *Journal of Applied Behavior Analysis*, 18(3), 201-214. Retrieved from http://search.proquest.com/docview/733478515?accountid=166958.
8. Shaikh, A.R., Yaroch, A.L., Nebeling, L., Yeh, M.C. and Resnicow, K.(2008). Psychosocial predictors of fruit and vegetable consumption in adults: a review of the literature. *American Journal of Preventative Medicine*. 34: 535–543.
9. Tudor-Locke, C., Myers, A. M., & Rodger, N. W. (2001). Development of a theory-based daily activity intervention for individuals with type 2 diabetes. *The Diabetes Educator*, 27(1), 85-93. Retrieved from http://search.proquest.com/docview/71299811?accountid=166958
10. Leahey, T.M and Wing, R.R. (2013). A randomized controlled pilot study testing three types of health coaches for obesity treatment: professional, peer, and mentor. *Obesity,* 21: 928–934. doi: 10.1038/oby.2012.179.
11. Gorin A, Phelan S. & Tate, D. et al. (2005). Involving support partners in obesity treatment. *Journal of Consulting & Clinical Psychology,* 73: 341–343.
12. Berino, J., Pintauro, S.J., Buzzell, P., et al. (2002). Does using the Internet facilitate the maintenance of weight

loss? *International Journal of Obesity*, 26(9):1254–1260.
13. Wilfley, D.E., Welch, R.R. Stein, R.I., et al. (2002). A randomized comparison of group cognitive-behavioral therapy and group interpersonal psychotherapy for the treatment of overweight individuals with binge-eating disorder. *Arch Gen Psychiatry*, 59: 713–721.
14. Wing, R.R.; Jeffery, R. W. (1999). Benefits of recruiting participants with friends and increasing social support for weight loss and maintenance. *Journal of Consulting and Clinical Psychology*, 67(1), 132-138. http://dx.doi.org/10.1037/0022-006X.67.1.132
15. Sampat, S., Kirschenbaum, D.S, Gierut, K.J., Germann, J.N.& Krawczyk, R. (2014). Ya gotta have friends: Social support and self-efficacy predict success following immersion treatment. *Obesity*, 22, (12), 2579–2585. DOI:10.1002/oby.20863.
16. Shimizu, M., Johnson, K., Wansink, B. (2014). In good company. The effect of an eating companion's appearance on food intake. *Appetite*, 83 (1), 263–268.
17. Christakis, N.A., Fowler, J.H. (2007). The spread of obesity in a large social network over 32 years. *New England Journal of Medicine*, 26, 357(4): 370-379.
18. Allen-o'donnell, M., Cottingham, M. D., Nowak, T. C., & Snyder, K. A. (2011). Impact of group settings and gender on meals purchased by college students. *Journal of Applied Social Psychology*, 41(9), 2268-2283. doi:http://dx.doi.org/10.1111/j.1559-1816.2011.00804.x
19. Christakis, N. A., & Fowler, J. H. (2007). The spread of obesity in a large social network over 32 years. *New England journal of medicine*, *357*(4), 370-379.
20. Siegel, D. J. (2006). An interpersonal neurobiology approach to psychotherapy. *Psychiatric Annals*, 36(4), 248-256. Retrieved from http://search.proquest.com/docview/217056447

Chapter 5: Stress Management for Weight Management

1. 1.Epel, E., Lapidus, R., McEwen, B., & Brownell, K. (2001). Stress may add bite to appetite in women: A laboratory study of stress-induced cortisol and eating behavior. *Psychoneuro- endocrinology*, 26(1), 37-49. Retrieved fromhttp://search.proquest. com/docview/ 70540379
2. Dallman, M. F., Pecoraro, N., Akana, S. F., Fleur, S. E., Gomez, F., Houshyar, H., . . . Manalo, S. (2003). Chronic stress and obesity: A new view of "comfort food". *Proceedings of the National Academy of Sciences,* USA, 100(20), 11696-11701. doi:http:// dx.doi.org/10.1073/pnas.1934666100
3. Ng, D.M. and Jeffery, R.W. (2003). Relationships between perceived stress and health behaviors in a sample of working adults. *Health Psychology*, 22, 638-642.
4. Takeda, E., Terao, J., Nakaya, Y., Miyamoto, K., Baba, Y. Chuman, H. 2004). Stress control and human nutrition, *Journal of Medical Invest*, 51, 139-145.
5. Kivimaki, M.J. Head, J., Ferrie, J.E., Shipley, M.J., Brunner, E.Vahtera, J.(2006). Work stress, weight gain and weight loss: evidence for bidirectional effects of job strain on body mass index in the Whitehall II study, *Int J Obesity*, 30, 982-987.
6. Kaplan, H.I. & Kaplan, H.S. (1957). The psychosomatic concept of obesity. *Journal of Mental and Nervous Disease,* 125, 181-201.
7. Laitinen, J., Ek, E., Sovio, U. (2002). Stress-related eating and drinking behavior and body mass index and predictors of this behavior, *Prev Med*, (34), 29-39 .
8. Levenstein, S.Rosenstock, S.Jacobsen, R.K. Jorgensen, T. 2015). Psychological Stress Increases Risk for Peptic Ulcer, Regardless of Helicobacter pylori Infection or Use of Non-steroidal Anti-inflammatory

Drugs. *Clinical Gastroenterology and Hepatology,* 13, (3), 498–506.e1.

9. Chang, L. (2011). The Role of Stress on Physiologic Responses and Clinical Symptoms in Irritable Bowel Syndrome *Gastroenterology*, 140, 3, 761–765.e5.
10. Huang et al. Kivimäki & Steptoe (2012). Stress and cardiovascular disease. *Cardiology,* 9, 360-370 | doi:10.1038/nrcardio.2012.45.
11. Manji, H.K. and Duman, R.S. (2001). Impairments of neuroplasticity and cellular resilience in severe mood disorders: implications for the development of novel therapeutics. *Psychopharmacol Bull*, 35: 5–49.
12. Foss, B., Sæterdal, L.R., Sindre M. and Dyrstad, S.M.(2014). Weight Reduction in Obese Correlates with Low Morning Cortisol Increase. *Journal of Exercise Physiology*, 17(3):70-76.
13. Epel, E., Lapidus, R., McEwen, B., & Brownell, K. (2001). Stress may add bite to appetite in women: A laboratory study of stress-induced cortisol and eating behavior. *Psychoneuro-endocrinology*, 26(1), 37-49.
14. Holt, S.H.A., Brand Miller, J. (1995). Increased insulin responses to ingested foods are associated with lessened satiety. *Appetite*, 24, (1), 43–54.
15. Björntorp, P. (2001). Do stress reactions cause abdominal obesity and comorbidities? *Obesity Reviews 2*(2), 73-86.
16. Schiewner, L.(1995). Mikronaehrstoffe und stress.*Vita Min Spur*, 10:11-15.
17. Groesz, L.M., McCoy, S, Carl, J., Saslow, L., Stewarta, J., Adlera, N., Laraiaa, B., Epela, E. (2012). What is eating you? Stress and the drive to eat. *Appetite*, 58 (2), 717–721
18. Loro, A.D., Orleans, C.S. (1981). Binge eating in obesity: preliminary findings and guidelines for behavioral analysis and treatment. *Addict Behav*, 6, 155–166.
19. Steptoe, A., Gibson, E. L., Vounonvirta, R., Williams, E. D., Hamer, M., Rycroft, J. A., . . . Wardle, J. (2007).

The effects of tea on psychophysiological stress responsivity and post-stress recovery: A randomised double-blind trial. *Psychopharmacology*, 190(1), 81-9. doi:http://dx.doi.org/10. 1007/s00213-006-0573-2

20. Yu, H., Chen, X., Liu, J., & Zhou, X. (2013). Gum chewing inhibits the sensory processing and the propagation of stress-related information in a brain network. PLoS One, 8(4) doi:http://dx.doi.org/10.1371/journal.pone.0057111
21. Lewis, D. (2009), Galaxy Stress Research, Mindlab International, Sussex University, UK
22. Kristeller, J.L. Hallett, C.B. 1999). An Exploratory Study of a Meditation-based Intervention for Binge Eating Disorder. *J Health Psychol*, 4, 3 357-363 doi: 10.1177/135910539900400305
23. Annells, S., Kho, K. and Bridge, P. (2015). Meditate don't medicate: how medical imaging evidence supports the role of meditation in the treatment of depression. Online. doi: 10.1016/j.radi.2015.08.002.
24. Linnemann, A., Ditzen, B., Strahler, J., Doerr, J. M., & Nater, U. M. (2015). Music listening as a means of stress reduction in daily life. *Psychoneuroendocrinology,* 60, 82-90. doi:http://dx.doi.org/10.1016/j.psyneuen.2015.06.008
25. Martin, R.A. and Lefcourt, H.M. (1983). Sense of humor as a moderator of the relation between stressors and moods. *Journal on Personality and Social Psychology,* 45:1313–24.
26. Berk, L.S., Tan, S.A., Fry, W.F, et al. (1989) Neuroendocrine and stress hormone changes during mirthful laughter. *American Journal of Medical Science*, 298:390–6.
27. Cousins, N. (1979). Anatomy of an Illness as Perceived by the Patient. Norton New York. ISBN 0-393-01252-2.
28. www.laughteryoga.org
29. www. yogaaustralia.org.au
30. Kristal, A. R., Littman, A. J., Benitez, D., & White, E. (2005). Yoga practice is associated with attenuated

weight gain in healthy, middle-aged men and women. *Alternative therapies in health and medicine*, 11(4), 28-33.

31. Light, K. C., Grewen, K. M., & Amico, J. A. (2005). More frequent partner hugs and higher oxytocin levels are linked to lower blood pressure and heart rate in premenopausal women. *Biological Psychology*, 69(1), 5-21. Retrieved from http://search.proquest.com/docview/67479639?accountid=166958
32. McConnell, A. R., Brown, C. M., Shoda, T. M., Stayton, L. E., & Martin, C. E. (2011). Friends with benefits: On the positive consequences of pet ownership. *Journal of Personality and Social Psychology*, 101(6), 1239-1252. doi:http://dx.doi.org/10.1037/a0024506 .
33. Iglesias, S.L., Azzara, S., Argibay, J.C., Arnaiz, M.L., de Valle Carpineta, M., Granchetti, H. & Lagomarsino, E.(2012). Psychological and Physiological Response of Students to Different Types of Stress Management Programs. *American Journal of Health Promotion*, 26, (6), 149-158.
34. Cox, T. L., Krukowski, R., Love, S. J., Eddings, K., DiCarlo, M., Chang, J. Y., . . . West, D. S. (2013). Stress management-augmented behavioral weight loss intervention for African American women: A pilot, randomized controlled trial. *Health Education & Behavior*, 40(1), 78-87. doi:http://dx.doi.org/10.1177/1090198112439411

Chapter 6: Forgiveness

1. 1.Hemmingsson, E., Johansson, K. & Reynisdottir, S.(2014). Effects of childhood abuse on adult obesity: a systematic review and meta-analysis. *Obesity Reviews*. DOI: 10.1111/obr.12216
2. Thoresen, C.E., Harris, A.H.S., & Luskin, F. (1999). Forgiveness and health: An unanswered question. In M.E. McCullough, K.I. Pargament, & C.E. Thoresen (Eds.). *Forgiveness: Theory, research, and practice* (pp. 254-280). New York: Guilford Press.

3. van Oyen Witvliet, C., Ludwig, T.E. and Van der Laan. K.L.(2001). Granting forgiveness or harboring grudges: Implications for Emotion, Physiology, and Health. *Psychological Science*, 12,(2), 117-123.
4. Baumeister, R.F., Exline, J.J. and Sommer, K L.(1998). The Victim Role, Grudge Theory, and Two Dimensions of Forgiveness. *Laws of life symposia series*, 1: 79-106.
5. Williams, R., & Williams, V. (1993). *Anger kills: Seventeen strategies for controlling the hostility that can harm your health*. New York: Harper Perennial.
6. van Oyen Witvliet, C., Ludwig, T.E. and Van der Laan. K.L.(2001). Granting forgiveness or harboring grudges: Implications for Emotion, Physiology, and Health. *Psychological Science*, 12,(2), 117-123.

Chapter 7: Sleep Away Your Fat

1. Taheri S, Lin L., Austin D., Young, T., Mignot, E. (2004) Short Sleep Duration Is Associated with Reduced Leptin, Elevated Ghrelin, and Increased Body Mass Index. PLoS Med 1(3): e62. doi:10.1371/journal.pmed.0010062
2. Reid, K. J., Santostasi, G., Baron, K. G., Wilson, J., Kang, J., & Zee, P. C. (2014). Timing and intensity of light correlate with body weight in adults. PLoS One, 9(4) doi:http://dx.doi.org/ 10.1371/journal.pone.0092251.
3. McFadden, E., Jones, M.E., Schoemaker, M.J., Ashworth, A. and Swerdlow, A.J. (2014). The Relationship Between Obesity and Exposure to Light at Night: Cross-Sectional Analyses of Over 100,000 Women in the Breakthrough Generations Study. *American Journal of Epidemiology.*, 180 (3): 245-250. doi: 10.1093/aje/kwu117.
4. Schmid, S. M., Hallschmid, M., Jauch-Chara, K., Born, J., & Schultes, B. (2008). A single night of sleep deprivation increases ghrelin levels and feelings of hunger in normal-weight healthy men. *Journal of*

Sleep Research, 17(3), 331-334. doi:http://dx.doi.org/10.1111/j.1365-2869.2008.00662.x

5. Aldabal, L., & Bahammam, A. S. (2011). Metabolic, endocrine, and immune consequences of sleep deprivation. *The Open Respiratory Medicine Journal*, 5, 31-43. doi:http://dx.doi.org/10.2174/1874306401105010031
6. 6.Brondel, L., Romer, M. A., Nougues, P. M., Touyarou, P., & Davenne, D. (2010). Acute partial sleep deprivation increases food intake in healthy men. *The American Journal of Clinical Nutrition*, 91(6), 1550-1559. doi:http://dx.doi.org/10.3945/ajcn.2009.28523.
7. Chamorro, R. A., Durán, S.,A., Reyes, S. C., Ponce, R., Algarín, C.,R., & Peirano, P. D. (2011). Sleep deprivation as a risk factor for obesity. *Revista Médica De Chile*, 139(7), 932-940. doi:http://dx.doi.org//S0034-98872011000700017.
8. American Psychiatric Association (2013). *Diagnostic & Statistical Manual of Mental Disorders* 5th edition. Washington, D.C. American Psychiatric Association.
9. Reas, D.L.& Grilo C.M. (2008).Review and meta-analysis of pharmacotherapy for binge-eating disorder. *Obesity (Silver Spring)* 16(9), 2024-2038
10. Cooper-Kazaz, R. (2012). Treatment of night eating syndromewithtopiramate:Dawnofanewday.doi:http://dx.doi.org/10.1097/JCP.0b013e31823f9051;doi:http://dx.doi.org/10.1007/s00394-011-0263-7.
11. Information adapated from www.apa.org helpcentre
12. Roehrs, T., and Roth, T. (2001). Sleep, Sleepiness, and Alcohol Use. National Institute on Alcohol Abuse and Alcoholism. Research and Health—pubs.niaaa.nih.gov.

Chapter 8: Get in the Mood for Weight Loss

1. Christensen, L. and Pettijohn, L.(2001). Mood and carbohydrate cravings. *Appetite*, 36(2), 137–145.

2. Rose, N., Koperski, S. & Golomb, B. A. (2010). Mood food: Chocolate and depressive symptoms in a cross-sectional analysis. *Archives of Internal Medicine*, 170(8), 699. Retrieved from http://search.proquest.com/docview/220079021? accountid=166958.
3. Macht, M. and Mueller, J. (2007). Immediate effects of chocolate on experimentally induced mood states, *Appetite*, 49(3), 667–674.
4. Klem, M.L. Wing, R., McGuire, M.T.; Seagle, H.M., Hill, J.O. (1998). Psychological symptoms in individuals successful at long-term maintenance of weight loss. *Health Psychology*, 17(4), 336-345. http://dx.doi.org/10.1037/0278-6133.17.4.336.
5. Pagoto, S., Bodenlos, J.S., Kantor, L., Gitkind,. M., Curtin, C. and Ma, Y. (2007). Association of Major Depression and Binge Eating Disorder with Weight Loss in a Clinical Setting. *Obesity*, 15 (11), 2557–2559. DOI:10.1038/oby.2007.307.
6. McElroy, S.L., Kotwal, R., Malhotra, S., Nelson, E.B., Keck, P.E. and Nemeroff, C.B. (2004). Are Mood Disorders and Obesity Related? A Review for the Mental Health Professional. *The Journal of Clinical Psychiatry*, 65: 634–651. doi:10.4088/jcp.v65n0507.
7. American Psychiatric Association (2013). *Diagnostic & Statistical Manual of Mental Disorders* 5th edition. Washington, D.C. American Psychiatric Association.
8. Sullivan, P.F., Neale MC, Kendler KS. (2000). Genetic epidemiology of major depression: review and meta-analysis. *Am J Psychiatry.*;157:1552–1562.
9. Kendler KS, Gardner CO, Prescott CA. (2006). Toward a comprehensive developmental model for major depression in men. *Am J Psychiatry*, 163:115–124.
10. Kendler, K.S., Gardner, C.O., Prescott, C.A. (2002). Toward a comprehensive developmental model for major depression in women. *Am J Psychiatry*, 159:1133–1145.
11. Walsh, A.E.S .(1995). *Journal of Affective Disorders*, 33, 89-97.

12. Anderson, I.M., Parry-Billings, M., Newsholme, E.A., Fairburn, C.G. & Cowen, P.J. (1990). Dieting reduces plasma tryptophan and alters brain 5HTP function in women. *Psychological Medicine*, 20:785-791.
13. Nishizawa, S., Benkelfat, C., Young, S. N., Leyton, M., Mzengeza, S., de Montigny, C., ... Diksic, M. (1997). Differences between males and females in rates of serotonin synthesis in human brain. Proceedings of the National Academy of Sciences of the United States of America, 94(10), 5308–5313.
14. Wurtman, R.J. and Wurtman, J.J. (1986). Carbohydrate craving, obesity and brain serotonin. *Appetite*, 7, 99-103.
15. Wurtman, R. J. and Wurtman, J. J. (1995), Brain Serotonin, Carbohydrate-Craving, Obesity and Depression. *Obesity Research*, 3:477S–480S. doi:10.1002/j.1550-8528.1995.tb00215.x.
16. Spring, B., Mailer, O., Wurtman, J., & Digman, L. (1983). Effects of protein and carbohydrate meals on mood and performance. *Journal of Psychiatric Research*, 17, 155-167.
17. Agras, W.S. and Telch, C.F. (*1998)*. The effects of caloric deprivation and negative affect on binge eating in obese binge-eating disordered women. *Behavior Therapy*, 29, 3, 491–503.
18. Wurtman, R. J. and Wurtman, J. J. (1995). Ibid
19. Wurtman, J., Wurtman, R., Mark, S., Tsay, R., Gilbert, W., Growdon, J. (1985). d-Fenfluramine Selectively Suppresses Carbohydrate Snacking by Obese Subjects. *International Journal of Eating Disorders*, 4(1), 89-99.
20. Baghai, T.C., Baldwin, D.S., Barret, B., Bauman, P., Ghalib, K. and Goodwin, G. (2007). Anti-depressant medications and other treatments for depressive disorders: a CINP taskforce report based on a review of the evidence. *International Journal of Neuropsychopharmacology*, 10 (1), S1-207.

21. Geddes et al. (2003) Relapse prevention with anti-depressant drug treatment in depressive disorders: a systematic review. *Lancet*, 361:653-61.
22. Darga, LL., Carroll-Michals, L, Botsford, S.J., and Lucas, C.P. (1991). Fluoxetine's effect on weight loss in obese subjects. *American Journal of Clinical Nutrition*, 54,(2), 321-325.
23. Goldstein, D.J. and Potvin, J.H.(1994). Long-term weight loss: the effect of pharmacologic agents. *American Journal Clinical Nutrition*, 60, (5), 647-657.
24. Rubinow, D.R., Su, T.(1997). Fluoxetine in the treatment of premenstrual dysphoria. *Neuropsychopharmacology*, 16, (5), 346–356.
25. Lopez, L.M., Kaptein, A.A, Helmerhorst, F.M. (2012) Oral contraceptives containing drospirenone for premenstrual syndrome. Cochrane Database of Systematic Reviews, 2. Art. No.: CD006586. DOI: 10.1002/14651858.CD006586.pub4.
26. Demyttenaere, K., Albert A, Mesters P, Dewé W, De Bruyckere K, Sangeleer M.J (2005). What happens with adverse events during 6 months of treatment with selective serotonin reuptake inhibitors? *Clinical Psychiatry*, 66 (7): 859-63.
27. Zimmermann, V., Kraus, T., Himmerich, H., et al. (2003) Epidemiology, implications and mechanisms underlying drug-induced weight gain in psychiatric patients. *J Psychiatr Res*, 37:193–220.
28. Finer, N. (1992). Serotoninergic system: Therapeutic implications in obesity. Acta Clinica Belgica. Supplementum, 14, 47-51. Retrieved from http://search.proquest.com/docview/ 73010433?accountid=166958
29. Reynolds, C. F., Butters, M. A., Lopez, O., Pollock, B. G., Dew, M. A., Mulsant, B. H., ... & Houck, P. R. (2011). Maintenance treatment of depression in old age: a randomized, double-blind, placebo-controlled evaluation of the efficacy and safety of donepezil combined with antidepressant pharmacotherapy. *Archives of general psychiatry*, *68*(1), 51-60.

30. Hollon, S.D. Stewart, M.O., Strunk, D. 2006). Enduring effects for cognitive behavior therapy in the treatment of depression and anxiety. *Annual Review of Psychology*, 57 (1), 285-315.DOI: 10.1146/annurev.psych.57.102904.190044
31. Evans, M. D., Hollon, S. D., DeRubeis, R. J., Piasecki, J. M., Grove, W. M., Garvey, M. J., & Tuason, V. B. (1992). Differential relapse following cognitive therapy and pharmacotherapy for depression. *Archives of General Psychiatry*, 49(10), 802-808. Retrieved from http://search. proquest.com/ docview/73288557?accountid=166958.
32. Hoes, M.J. (1982). L-tryptophan in depression. *Journal of Orthomolecular Psychiatry*, 4:231.
33. Young, S.N. (2007). Folate and depression–a neglected problem. *Journal of Psychiatry Neuroscience*, 32(2): 80-82.
34. Coppen, A. (2005). Treatment of depression: time to consider folic acid and vitamin B12. *Journal of Psychopharmacology,* 19, (1), 59-65 doi: 10.1177/0269881105048899.
35. Taylor, M.J., Carney, S. Geddes, J. and Goodwin, G. (2003). Cochrane Database of Systematic Reviews, 2.
36. Gorgojo Martínez, J.J., Ruiz, F.A. & Candil, S.D. (2006). Baseline serum folate level may be a predictive factor of weight loss in a morbid-obesity-management programme. *British Journal of Nutrition*, 96 (05), 956-964. DOI: http://dx.doi.org/10.1017/BJN20061899
37. Eby, G.A. and Eby, K.L. (2006). Rapid recovery from major depression using magnesium treatment. *Med Hypotheses*, 67(2): 362-370.
38. Appleton, K.M., Rogers, P.J. and Ness, A.R. (2010). Updated systematic review and meta-analysis of the effects of n−3 long-chain polyunsaturated fatty acids on depressed mood. *American Society for Nutrition*, 1-14. doi: 10.3945/ajcn.2009.28313.

39. Morgan, A.J. Jorm, A.F. (2008). Self help interventions for depressive disorders and depressive symptoms: a systematic review. *Annals of General Psychiatry*, 17, 13.
40. Rebouche, C.J. (1999). Carnitine. In: *Modern Nutrition in Health and Disease*, 9th Edition (edited by Shils M.E., Olson J.A, Shike M, Ross, AC). Lippincott Williams and Wilkins, New York, pp. 505-12.
41. Shaw, K., Turner, J., Del, M.C. (2002). Tryptophan and 5-HTP for depression. Cochrane Database of Systematic Reviews, 1. Art no CD003198.doi:10.1002/14651858.CD003198.
42. 39.Cangiano, C., Avano A. L. & Del, B. M. (1998). Effects of oral 5-hydroxytryptophan on energy intake and macronutrient selection in non-insulin dependent diabetic patients. *International Journal of Obesity Related Metabolism Disorders*, 22, 648-54.
43. Cangiano, C., Ceci, F., Cascino, A. (1992). Eating behaviour and adherence to dietary prescriptions in obese adult subjects treated with 5-hydroxytryptophan. *American Journal of Clinical Nutrition*, 56:863-867.
44. umm.edu/health/medical/altmed/supplement/5hydroxytryptophan-5htp
45. Szegedi, A., Kohnen, R., Dienel, A. & Kieser, M. (2005) Acute treatment of moderate to severe depression with hypericum extract WS 5570 (St John's wort): Randomised controlled double-blind non-inferiority trial versus paroxetine. *BMJ*, 330: 503.
46. www.nlm.nih.gov/medlineplus/druginfo/natural/329.html
47. Coulter, M.L.I., Morton, S.C., Favreau, J., Venuturupalli, S., Chiappelli, F., Rossi, F., Orshansky, G. Jungvig, L.K., Roth, E.A.Suttorp, M.J.and Shekelle, P.S (2003). S-Adenosyl-L-Methionine (SAMe) for Treatment of Depression, Osteoarthritis, and Liver Disease: Summary National Institutes of Health.

48. Sarris, J., Papakostas, G.I.Vitolo, O., Fava, M., Mischoulon, D. (2014). S-adenosyl methionine (SAMe) versus escitalopram and placebo in major depression RCT: Efficacy and effects of histamine and carnitine as moderators of response. *Journal of Affective Disorders*, 164, 76–81 doi.org/10.1016/j.jad.2014.03.041
49. van Die M., Burger, H.G., Teede, H.J., Bon, K.M. 2013). Vitex agnus-castus extracts for female reproductive disorders. A systematic review of clinical trials. *Planta Med*; 79: 562–575. DOI:10.1055/s-0032-1327831.
50. Stanton, R. and Reaburn,P. (2014). Exercise and the treatment of depression: A review of the exercise program. *Journal of Science and Medicine in Sport*, 17, 2, 177–182.
51. Lewy, A.J, Emens, J.S., Songer, J.B., Sims, N., Laurie, A.L., Fiala, S.C. & Buti, A.L. (2009). Winter Depression: Integrating mood, circadian rhythms, and the sleep/wake and light/dark cycles into a bio-psycho-socialenvironmental model. *Sleep Med Clin.*, 4: 285-99.
52. Boyce, P. and Barriball, E. (2010). Circadian rhythms and depression. *Aust Fam Physician.*; 39: 307-10
53. Roecklein, K.A, Rohan, K.J., and Postolache, T.T. (2010). Is seasonal affective disorder a bipolar variant? *Curr Psychiatr.* 9: 42-54.
54. Virk, G., Reeves, G., Rosenthal, N.E., Sher, L. & Postolache, T.T. (2009). Short exposure to light treatment improves depression scores in patients with seasonal affective disorder: A brief report. *Int J Disabil Hum Dev.*, 8: 283-86.
55. Penckofer, S., Kouba, J., Byrn, M. & Estwing, F.C. (2010). Vitamin D and depression: where is all the sunshine? *Issues Ment Health Nurs.*, 31: 385-93
56. Berk, M., Sanders, K.M., Pasco, J.A., Jacka, F.N., Williams, L.J., Hayles, A.L. & Dodd, S. (2007). Vitamin D deficiency may play a role in depression. *Med Hypotheses.*, 69: 1316-9.

57. Alpayci, M., Ozdemir, O., Erdem, S., Bozan, N., & Yazmalar, L. (2012). Sunglasses may play a role in depression. *Journal of Mood Disorders*, 2(2), 80. doi:http://dx.doi.org/10.5455/jmood.20120529055051.
58. Morgan, A. J., & Jorm, A. F. (2008). Self-help interventions for depressive disorders and depressive symptoms: A systematic review. *Annals of General Psychiatry*, *7*, 13. doi:http://dx.doi.org/10.1186/1744-859X-7-13

Chapter 9: Body Image: Love Your Body

1. Friedman, K.E., Reichmann, S.K., Costanzo, P.R. & Musante, G.J. (2002). Body image partially mediates the relationship between obesity and psychological distress. *Obesity Res.*,10:33– 41
2. Herbert, A., Gerry, N.P, McQueen, M.B, Heid, I.M., Pfeufer, A., Illig, T., Wichmann, H.E., Meitinger, T., Hunter, D., Hu, F.B., Colditz, G., Hinney, A., Hebebrand, J., Koberwitz, K., Zhu, X., Cooper, R., Ardlie, K., Lyon, H, Hirschhorn, J.N., Laird, N.M., Lenburg, M.E., Lange, C., Christman, M.F. (2006). A common genetic variant is associated with adult and childhood obesity. *Science*, 312(5771), 279-83.
3. Maes, H.H.M., Neale, M.C. and Eaves, L.J. (1997). Genetic and Environmental Factors in Relative Body Weight and Human Adiposity. *Behavior Genetics*, 27, (4), 325-351.
4. Loos, R. J. F., & Bouchard, C. (2008). FTO: the first gene contributing to common forms of human obesity. *Obesity Reviews*, 9(3), 246-250.
5. Corella, D., Peloso, G, Arnett D.K., Demissie S, Cupples, L.A., Tucker, K., Lai, C.Q., Parnell, L.D., Coltell, O., Lee, Y.C., Ordovas, J.M. (2009). APOA2, dietary fat, and body mass index: replication of a gene-diet interaction in 3 independent populations. *Arch Intern Medicine*;169(20):1897-906. doi: 10.1001/archinternmed.2009.343.

6. Kilpeläinen, T.O., Qi, L., Brage, S., et al. (2011). Physical activity attenuates the influence of FTO variants on obesity risk: a meta-analysis of 218,166 adults and 19,268 children.;8:e1001116. Epub.
7. Ricca, V., Castellini, G., Mannucci, E., Lo Sauro, C., Ravaldi, C. et al., (2010): Comparison of individual and group cognitive behavioral therapy for binge eating disorder. A randomized, three-year follow-up study. *Appetite*, 55(3), 656-665.
8. Song, A. Y., Rubin, J. P., Thomas, V., Dudas, J. R., Marra, K. G., & Fernstrom, M. H. (2006). Body image and quality of life in post massive weight loss body contouring patients. *Obesity*, 14(9), 1626-36. doi:http://dx.doi.org/10.1038/oby.2006.187
9. Pecori, L., Cervetti, G. G., Serra, Marinari, G. M., Migliori, F., & Adami, G. F. (2007). Attitudes of morbidly obese patients to weight loss and body image following bariatric surgery and body contouring. *Obesity Surgery*, 17(1), 68-73. doi:http://dx.doi.org/10.1007/s11695-007-9008-3.
10. Carraça, E.,V., Silva, M. N., Markland, D., Vieira, P. N., Minderico, C. S., Sardinha, L. B., & Teixeira, P. J. (2011). Body image change and improved eating self-regulation in a weight management intervention in women. *The International Journal of Behavioral Nutrition and Physical Activity*, 8, 75. doi:http://dx.doi.org/10.1186/1479-5868-8-75
11. Marcus, M.D. (1997). Adapting Treatment for Patients with Binge Eating Disorder. D.M. Garner & P.E. Garfinkel (Eds). *Handbook of Treatment for Eating Disorders* (2nd Ed). The Guilford Press. New York.
12. Thompson, J.K. & Stice, E (2001). Thin ideal internalization: mounting evidence for a new risk factor for body image disturbance ad eating pathology. *Current Direction in Psychological Science*, 10, 181-183.
13. Flegal, K.M., Graubard, B.I., Williamson, D.F. and Gail, M.H. (2005) Excess deaths associated with

underweight, overweight, and obesity. *Journal of the American Medical Association*, 293(15): 1861–1867.
14. Lee, C.D., Blair, S.N. & Jackson, A.S. (1999). Cardiorespiratory fitness, body composition, and all-cause and cardiovascular disease mortality in men. *American Journal Clinical Nutrition*, 69: 373–380.
15. Hayes, L., Pearce, M.S., Firbank, M.J.,Walker, M., Taylor, R. and Unwin, N.C. (2010). Do obese but metabolically normal women differ in intra-abdominal fat and physical activity levels from those with the expected metabolic abnormalities? A cross-sectional study. *BMC. Public Health*, 10: 723.
16. Brown, R.E. & Kuk, J.L. (2014). Consequences of obesity and weight loss: a devil's advocate position. *Obesity Reviews*. doi: 10.1111/obr.12232
17. Li, S., Zhao, J.H., Luan, J., Ekelund, U., Luben, R.N. and Khaw K-T, et al. (2010). Physical Activity Attenuates the Genetic Predisposition to Obesity in 20,000 Men and Women from EPIC-Norfolk Prospective Population Study. PLoS Med 7(8): e1000332. doi:10.1371/journal.pmed.1000332.
18. Thompson P.D., Crouse, S.F., Goodpaster, B., Kelley, D., Moyna, N. and Pescatello, L. (2001). The acute versus the chronic response to exercise. *Medical Science Sports Exercise*; 33(6): S438–S445. discussion S452–3.).
19. Rosen, J.C. (1997). *Cognitive Behavioral Body Image Therapy. In Handbook of Treatment of Eating Disorders*. D. M Garner & P. E. Garfinkel. The Guilford Press. New York.
20. Jackson, S.E., Steptoe, A., Beeken, R.J., Kivimaki M. and Wardle, J. (2014). Psychological Changes following Weight Loss in Overweight and Obese Adults: A Prospective Cohort Study. PLoS ONE 9(8): e104552. doi:10.1371/journal.pone.0104552
21. Brickman, P., Coates, D. & Janoff-Bulman, R. (1978). Lottery winners and accident victims: is happiness

relative? *Journal of Personality and Social Psychology*, 36(8): 917-27.
22. Ogden, J. (1992). *Fat chance! The Myth of Dieting Explained.* New York: Routledge.

Chapter 10: How to Overcome Food Addiction, Binge Eating, and Emotional Eating

1. Elfhag, K. and Rössner, S. (2005). Who succeeds in maintaining weight loss? A conceptual review of factors associated with weight loss maintenance and weight regain. *Obesity Reviews*, 6, (1) 67–85.
2. Wing, R.R. and Phelan, S. (2005). Long-term weight loss maintenance. *American Journal of Clinical*
3. *Nutrition*, 82, 1 222S-225S.
4. Pagoto, S., Bodenlos, J.S., Kantor, L., Gitkind,. M., Curtin, C. and Ma, Y. (2007). Association of Major. Depression and Binge Eating Disorder with Weight Loss in a Clinical Setting. *Obesity*, 15 (11), 2557–2559. DOI:10.1038/oby.2007.307
5. Yamamoto, T. (2003). Brain Mechanisms of sweetness and palatability of sugars. *Nutrition Reviews*. 61(5.2): S5-9.
6. Pelchat, M.L. (2002). Of human bondage: food craving, obsession, compulsion and addiction.
7. *Physiology and Behaviour*. 76 (3):347-52.
8. American Psychiatric Association (2013). *Diagnostic & Statistical Manual of Mental Disorders*(5th edition). Washington, D.C. American Psychiatric Association.
9. Hamburger, W W(1957). Psychological aspects of obesity. *Bulletin of the New York Academy of*
10. *Medicine*, 33,(11), 771-782.
11. Kaye, W.H. Jimerson, D.C., Lake. C.R and Ebert, M.H. (1985). Altered norepinephrine metabolism following long term weight recovery in patients with anorexia nervosa. *Psychiatry Research*, 14 (4), 333-342.
12. Marney, A., White, Carlos M. and Grilo, (2005). Psychometric properties of the Food Craving

Inventory among obese patients with binge eating disorder. *Eating Behaviors*, 6 (3), 239–245
13. Barry, D., Clarke, M. and Petry, N.M. (2009).Obesity and its relationship to addictions: is overeating a form of addictive behavior? *The American Journal on Addictions*, 18.6: 439-451.
14. Del Parigi, A., Chen, K., Salbe, A.D; Reiman, E.M. and Tataranni, P. A.(2003). Are We Addicted to Food? *Obesity Research*, 11(4) 493-495.
15. Volkow, N.D, Wang, G.J., Maynard, L., et al. (2003). Brain dopamine is associated with eating behaviors in humans. *International Journal of Eating Disorders*, 33, 136.
16. Barry, D., & Petry, N. M. (2009). Obesity and psychiatric disorders. *Psychiatric Times, 26*(12), 49-57. Retrieved from http://search.proquest.com/docview/204590333?accountid=166958
17. receptors) and say it leads people to engage compulsively in rewarding behaviors such as drug use and eating
18. Abizaid, A., Gao, Q. & Horvath, T.L; (2006): Thoughts for food: brain mechanisms and peripheral energy balance. *Neuron*, 51(6), 691-702.
19. Drewnowski, A., Gosnell, B., Klahn, D. D. & Canum, K.. (1989). Sensory preferences for sugar and fat: Evidence for opioid involvement. *Appetite*, 12, 206.
20. Blundell, J.E., Stubbs, R.J., Goldinga, C., Crodena, F., Alama, R., Whybrowb, S., Le Nourya, J.
21. Lawtona, C.L. (2005). Resistance and susceptibility to weight gain: Individual variability in response to a high-fat diet. *Physiology & Behavior*, 86, (5), 614–622
22. American Psychiatric Association (2013). *Diagnostic & Statistical Manual of Mental* Disorders 5th edition. Washington, D.C. American Psychiatric Association.
23. 17.Goldschmidt, A. B., Hilbert, A., Manwaring, J. L., Wilfley, D. E., Pike, K. M., Fairburn, C. G.,...Striegel-Moore, R.H. (2010). The significance of overvaluation of shape and weight in binge eating disorder. *Behaviour Research and Therapy*, 48, 187–193.

24. Grilo, C.M., Hrabosky, J. I., & White, M. A. (2008). Overvaluation of shape and weight in binge eating disorder and overweight controls: Refinement of a diagnostic construct. *Journal of Abnormal Psychology,* 117, 414–419.
25. Ahrberg, M., Trojca, D., Nasrawi, N.,Vocks, S. (2011). Body Image Disturbance in Binge Eating Disorder: A Review. *European Eating Disorders Review*, 19(5), 375–381. DOI:10.1002/erv.1100
26. Stunkard, A.(2002). Binge-eating Disorder and the Night Eating Syndrome. In: Fairburn C., Brownell K. (Eds.), *Eating Disorders and Obesity: A Comprehensive Handbook*. New York, Guilford Press, 107-121.
27. Fairburn, C.G., Doll, H. A., Welch, S. L.& Hay, P.(1998). Risk factors for BED: A community-based, case-control study. *Journal of Archives of General Psychiatry*. 55.5: 425-32.
28. Hemmingsson, E., Johansson, K. & Reynisdottir, S.(2014). Effects of childhood abuse on adult
29. obesity: a systematic review and meta-analysis. *Obesity Reviews*. DOI: 10.1111/obr.12216
30. Grant, P.G. & Boersma, H. (2005). Making sense of being fat: A hermeneutic analysis of adults' explanations for obesity. *Counselling and Psychotherapy Research* (5), 3, 212-220. DOI: 10.1080/17441690500310429
31. Herman, C. P., & Polivy, J. (1988). Excess and restraint in bulimia. In K.Pirke,W.Vandereycken, & D. Ploog (Eds.), *The psychobiology of bulimia* (pp. 33-41). Munich: Springer Verlag.
32. Geliebter, A. & Aversa, A. (2003). Emotional eating in over-weight, normal weight, and underweight individuals. *Eating Behaviour*, 3: 341–7.
33. Ganley, R.M. (1989). Emotion and eating in obesity. A review of the literature. *International Journal of Eating Disorders*, 8: 343–61.
34. Schulz, S. and Laessle, R.G. 2012). Stress-induced laboratory eating behavior in obese women with binge eating disorder. *Appetite*, 58 (2), 457–461.

35. Festinger, David S., Rubenstein, David F., Marlowe, Douglas B.; Platt, Jerome J. (2001). Relapse: Contributing factors, causative models, and empirical considerations. In Relapse and recovery in addictions, by Tims, Frank M. (Ed); Leukefeld, Carl G. (Ed); Platt, Jerome J. (Ed), 122-142. New Haven, CT, US:Yale University Press.
36. Grilo, Shiffman & Wing, 1989; Sarlio-Lahteenkorva, (1998) Appetite. eat in response to happy mood.
37. Isnard, P., Michel, G., Frelut, M.-L., Vila, G., Falissard, B., Naja, W., Navarro, J. and Mouren-Simeoni, M.-C. (2003), Binge eating and psychopathology in severely obese adolescents. *Int. J. Eat. Disord.*, 34: 235–243. doi:10.1002/eat.10178
38. Isnard et al. (2003). Ibid.
39. Timmerman, G.M. &Acton, G.J. (2001). the relationship between basic need satisfaction and emotional eating. *Issues in Mental Health Nursing,* 22, 7, 691-701 DOI:10.1080/01612840119628
40. Kaplan, H.I. & Kaplan, H.S. (1957). The psychosomatic concept of obesity. *Journal of Mental and Nervous Disease*, 125, 181-201.
41. Bohon, C., Stice, E. and Spoor, S. (2009). Female emotional eaters show abnormalities in consummatory and anticipatory food reward: a functional magnetic resonance imaging study. *International Journal of Eating Disorders*, 42, 210–221.
42. Hetherington, M.M., MacDiarmid, J.L. (1993). Chocolate addiction: a preliminary study of its description and its relationship to problem eating. *Appetite*, 21: 233–246.
43. Wansink, B., Cheney, M.M., Chan N. (2003). Exploring comfort food preferences across age and gender. *Physiological Behaviour*, 79: 739–47.
44. Bruch, H. (1973). *Eating Disorders.* Obesity and Anorexia Nervosa. Riverside, CA: Behavior Science Book Service.

45. van Strien T. (2000). Ice-cream consumption, tendency toward overeating, and personality. *Int J Eat Disorders*, 28(4):460-4.
46. The Australian Longitudinal Study on Women's Health. (1996). Universities of Newcastle and Queensland.
47. Mellin, L., Croughan-Minihane, M., Dickey, L.(1997) The Solution Method: 2 year trends in weight, blood pressure, exercise, depression, and functioning of adults trained in development skills. *Journal of the American Dietetic Association*, 97:1133-1138.

Chapter 11: Forbidden Fruit - How to Eat Your Favourite Food

1. Kuijer, R.G. & Boyce, J.A (2014). Chocolate cake. Guilt or celebration? Associations with healthy eating attitudes, perceived behavioural control, intentions and weight-loss. Appetite, 74, 48–54. doi:10.1016/j.appet.2013.11.013.
2. Lemmens, S.G., Born, J.M., Rutters, F., Schoffelen, P.F., Wouters, L. and Westerterp-Plantenga, M.S. (2010). Dietary Restraint and Control Over "Wanting" Following Consumption of "Forbidden" Food. Obesity, 18, (10), 1926–1931, DOI:10.1038/oby.2010.36.
3. Stirling. L.J. and Yeomans, M.R. (2004). Effect of exposure to a forbidden food on eating in restrained and unrestrained women. International Journal of Eating Disorders, 35 (1), 59–68, DOI:10.1002/eat.10232.
4. Parker, Gordon et al.(2006).Mood state effects of chocolate. Journal of Affective Disorders, 92 (2), 149—159.
5. Macht, M. & Mueller J. (2007). Immediate effects of chocolate on experimentally induced mood states. *Appetite*, 49: 667–74.
6. Davis, J.M., Lowy, M.T., Yim, G.K, Lamb, D.R & Malven, P.V. (1983). Relationships between plasma

concentrations of immunocreactive beta-endorphin and food intake in rats. Peptides, 4:79–83.
7. Mechoulam, R., Berry, E.M., Avraham, Y., Di Marzo, V., Fride, E.(2006). Endocannabinoids, feeding and suckling - from our perspective. *International Journal of Obesity*, 30: S24–8.
8. Morewedge, C.K., Huh, Y.E. & Vosgerau, J. (2010). Thought for food: imagined consumption reduces actual consumption. Science, 10; 330(6010):1530-3.

Chapter 12: Hypnosis: When the Pendulum Swings, Change Begins

1. http://www.historyofhypnosis.org/franz-anton-mesmer/
2. Eisen, M.R. (1993). Psychoanalytic and Psychodynamic Models of Hypnoanalysis. In Rue, Lynn & Kirsch. Handbook of Clinical Hypnosis. APA, Washington
3. Markham, U. (1985). Hypnothink. Northhamptonshire. Thorsons.
4. Ranganathan, V.K., Siemionow, V., Liu, J.Z., Sahgal, V., Yue, G.H. (2004). From mental power to muscle power--gaining strength by using the mind. Neuropsychologia. 42(7): 944-56.
5. Kappes, H.B. & Oettingen, G. (2011) Positive fantasies about idealized futures sap energy
6. *Journal of Experimental Social Psychology*, 47, (4), 719–729.
7. Thompson, J.K. & Stice, E (2001). Thin ideal internalization: mounting evidence for a new risk factor for body image disturbance ad eating pathology. Current Direction in Psychological Science, 10, 181-183.
8. Littleton H.L., Ollendick, T. (2003) Negative body image and disordered eating behavior in children and adolescents: What places youth at risk and how can these problems be prevented? *Clin Child Fam* Psychol Rev, 6(1):51–66

9. Klopfer, B. (1957). Psychological variables in Human cancer. Journal of Projective Techniques, 21, 331-340.
10. Crum, A.J, Corbin, W.R., Brownell, K.D., Salovey, P. (2011). Mind over milkshakes: mindsets, not just nutrients, determine ghrelin response. Health Psychology, 30(4):424-9. doi: 10.1037/a0023467
11. Emoto, M. The Hidden Messages of Water. www.masaru-emoto.net/english/water-crystal.html
12. Andersen, M.S. (1985). Hypnotizability as a factor in the hypnotic treatment of obesity. International Journal of Clinical and Experimental Hypnosis, 33, 150-159.
13. Kirsch, I. (1985). Response expectancy as a determinant of experience and behavior. American Psychologist, 40, 1189-1202.
14. Gfeller, J.D., Lynn, S.J. & Pribble, W.E. (1987). Enhancing hypnotic susceptibility: Interpersonal and rapport factors. *Journal of Personality and Social Psychology*, 52, 586-595.
15. Allison, D.B. & Faith, M.S. (1996). Hypnosis as an adjunct to cognitive-behavioral psychotherapy for obesity: a meta-analytical reappraisal. *J Consult Clin Psychol*; 64: 513–516.
16. 14.Mendoza, M. E., & Capafons, A. (2009). Efficacy of clinical hypnosis: A summary of its empirical evidence. Papeles del Psicólogo, 30(2), 98-116.
17. Johnson, D. (1997). Weight loss for women: studies of smokers and nonsmokers using hypnosis and multicomponent treatments with and without overt aversion. Psychological Reports, 80, 931-933. doi: 10.2466/pr0.1997.80.3.931
18. Kirsch, I., Montgomery, G and Sapirstein, G. (1995). Hypnosis as an adjunct to cognitive-behavioral psychotherapy: A meta-analysis. *Journal of Consulting and Clinical Psychology*, 63(2), 214-220. http://dx.doi.org/10.1037/0022-006X.63.2.214.
19. ABC TV science program 'Catalyst', Paul Willis.
20. Postel, T. (2013). Childbirth climax: The revealing of obstetrical orgasm. Sexologies, 22, 4, e89–e92.

Chapter 13: Psychological Therapy—the Diet for the Mind

1. Blackburn, I.M., Bishop, S., Glen, A.I., Whalley, L.J. & Christie, J.E. (1981).The efficacy of cognitive therapy in depression: a treatment trial using cognitive therapy and pharmacotherapy, each alone and in combination. *The British Journal of Psychiatry*, 139 (3) 181-189; DOI: 10.1192/bjp.139.3.181
2. Hartmann-Boyce, J., Johns, D.J., Jebb, S.A. & Aveyard, P. (2014.) Effect of behavioural techniques and delivery mode on effectiveness of weight management: systematic review, meta-analysis and meta-regression. *Obesity Reviews*, 15 (7), 598–609.
3. Vocks, S.,Tuschen-Caffier, B., Pietrowsky, R., Rustenbach, S.J., Kersting, A., Herpertz, S.(2009). Meta-analysis of the effectiveness of psychological and pharmacological treatments for binge eating disorder. *International Journal of Eating Disorders*, 43, (3), 205–217.DOI:10.1002/eat.20696
4. Brauhardt, A., de Zwaan, M., Hilbert, A. (2014). The therapeutic process in psychological treatments for eating disorders: a systematic review. *The International Journal of Eating Disorders*, 47(6): 565-584.
5. Wilson, G.T., Wilfley, D.E., Agras, S.W.& Bryson, S.W. (2010). Psychological Treatments of Binge Eating Disorder. *Archives of General Psychiatry*. 67(1):94-101. doi:10.1001/archgenpsychiatry.170.
6. Seligman.M.E.P. (1995). American Psychologist The effectiveness of psychotherapy: The Consumer Reports study. *American Psychologist*, 50(12), 965-974. http://dx.doi.org/10.1037/0003-066X.50.12.965
7. Grilo, C. M, White, M. A., Wilson, G. T., Gueorguieva, R., Masheb, R. M. (2012). Rapid response predicts 12-month post-treatment outcomes in binge-eating disorder: theoretical and clinical implications. *Psychological Medicine*, 42.4, 807-17.
8. Peterson, C. B, Mitchell, J. E., Crow, S. J, Crosby, R.D, & Wonderlich, S. A. (2009). The Efficacy of Self-Help

Group Treatment and Therapist-Led Group Treatment for Binge Eating Disorder. *American Journal of Psychiatry*, 166.12: 1347-54.

9. Butler, A.C., Chapman, J.E., Forman, E.M. and Beck, A.T. (2006). The empirical status of cognitive-behavioral therapy: A review of meta-analyses. *Clinical Psychology Review*, 26, (1), 17–31.
10. Marcus, M. (1997). *Handbook of Treatment for Eating Disorders* 2nd edition. in Garner & Garfinkel. P 484-493. Adapting Treatment for Patients with Binge Eating Disorder.
11. Medina, J. H., Bekinschteina, P., Cammarota, M. and Izquierdo I.(2008). Do memories consolidate to persist or do they persist to consolidate? *Behavioural Brain Research*, 192 (1), 1, 61–69. Biobehavioural Plasticity
12. Bambling, M .(2014). *Psychotherapy in Australia*, 20, 2, 4-8.
13. Wilfley, D.E., Welch, R.R., Stein, R.I, et al. (2002). A randomized comparison of group cognitive-behavioral therapy and group interpersonal psychotherapy for the treatment of overweight individuals with binge-eating disorder. *Arch Gen Psychiatry*, 59:713–721.
14. Ricca, V., Castellini, G., Mannucci, E., Lo Sauro, C., Ravaldi, C. et al., (2010): Comparison of individual and group cognitive behavioral therapy for binge eating disorder. A randomized, three-year follow-up study, *Appetite*, 55.3 656-665.

Chapter 14: EMDR

1. Vocks, S., Tuschen-Caffier, B., Pietrowsky, R., Rustenbach, S. J., Kersting, A. and Herpertz, S. (2010), Meta-analysis of the effectiveness of psychological and pharmacological treatments for binge eating disorder. Int. *J. Eat. Disord.*, 43: 205–217. doi: 10.1002/eat.20696

2. Shapiro, F. (2001). *Eye movement desensitisation and reprocessing*: basic principles, protocols, and procedures (2nd ed). New York: Guilford Press.
3. www.emdr.com
4. Balbo, M. (May 2003). EMDR treatment of binge eating disorders. Symposium conducted at the annual meeting of the EMDR Europe Association, Rome, Italy.
5. Hornsfeld, H. (June 2005). Cue exposure and EMDR: a new protocol description of procedure and demonstration of clinical application in the treatment of binge eating. In EMDR and Eating Disorders. Symposium conducted at the annual meeting of the EMDR Europe Association, Brussels, Belgium.
6. www.australianbreathworkassociation.org.au
7. www.drweil.com
8. Eyerman, J. (2013). Clinical Report of Holotropic Breathwork in 11,000 Psychiatric Inpatients in a Community Hospital Setting. MAPS Bulletin Special Edition. - metslesvoiles.org
9. Ruden, R.A.(2005) Neurobiological basis for the observed peripheral sensory modulation of emotional responses. *Traumatology*. 11:145Y158.
10. Trubo, R. Callahan, R. (2001). Tapping the healer within: using thought field therapy to instantly conquer your fears, anxieties, and emotional distress. Chicago, Ill: Contemporary Books. ISBN0-8092-9880-5.
11. Craig, G. (1999) *Emotional freedom techniques:* The manual. The Sea Ranch, California: Author.
12. Johnson, C., Shala, M., Sejdijaj, X., Odell, R., & Dabishevci, K. (2001). Thought field therapy-soothing the bad moments of Kosovo. *Journal of Clinical Psychology, 57*(10), 1237-1240. Retrieved from http://search.proquest.com/docview/71129129?accountid=166958
13. Treatment of Food Cravings in Overweight and Obese Adults: A Comparison of Emotional Freedom Techniques and Cognitive Behavioural Therapy with

12-month follow-up. Eating Disorders and Obesity Conference, 26th -27 May 2014, Gold Coast

14. Bachelor, A. Horvath, A., Hubble, M.A. (Ed); Duncan, Barry L. (Ed); Miller, Scott D. (Ed), (1999). The therapeutic relationship. *The heart and soul of change: What works in therapy* (pp. 133-178). Washington, DC, US: American Psychological Association, xxiv, 462 pp. http://dx.doi.org/10.1037/11132-004
15. Scott, L., Martinovich, Zoran, Lutz, Wolfgang, Lyons, John S. (2005). The effect of therapist experience on psychotherapy outcomes. *Clinical Psychology and Psychotherapy*, 12.6
16. 16.McKay, K.M., Zac E. Imel, Bruce E. Wampold. (2006). Psychiatrist effects in the psycho-pharmacological treatment of depression. *Journal of Affective Disorders*, 92, Issues 2–3, 287–290doi:10.1016/j.jad.2006.01.020
17. Heinonen, E., Lindfors, Olavi; Laaksonen, Maarit A; Knekt, P. 2012). Therapists' professional and personal characteristics as predictors of outcome in short- and long-term psychotherapy. *Journal of Affective Disorders*138.3 : 301-312.

Chapter 15: Diet

1. bodyandsoul.com.au: Ricki-Lee Coulter on getting fit
2. womansday.com.au: Kate Ritchie: how I got my best body ever
3. au.tv.yahoo.com/sunrise: diet that changed Kerri-Anne's body
4. dailymail.co.uk/.../Melissa Doyle
5. aww.com.au: Julia Morris
6. Dombrowski, S.U., Knittle, K., Avenell A, Araújo-Soares V, Sniehotta, F. F. (2014). Long term maintenance of weight loss with non-surgical interventions in obese adults: systematic review and meta-analyses of randomised controlled trials. *British Medical Journal*, 348. doi:http: //dx.doi.org/10.1136 /bmj.g2646;348:g2646

7. Franz, M. J., Van Wormer, J. J., Crain, A. L., Boucher, J. L., Histon, T., Caplan, W., ... & Pronk, N. P. (2007). Weight-loss outcomes: a systematic review and meta-analysis of weight-loss clinical trials with a minimum 1-year follow-up. *Journal of the American Dietetic Association*, *107*(10), 1755-1767.
8. Curioni, C. C., & Lourenco, P. M. (2005). Long-term weight loss after diet and exercise: a systematic review. *International journal of obesity*, *29*(10), 1168-1174.
9. Chapman, C. D., Benedict, C., Brooks, S. J., & Schiöth, H.B. (2012). Lifestyle determinants of the drive to eat: A meta-analysis. The American Journal of Clinical Nutrition, 96(3), 492-497. doi:http://dx.doi.org/10.3945/ajcn.112.039750
10. Obesity guidelines. Obesity Journal (2014).
11. Sacks, F.M., Bray, G.A., Carey, V.J. (2009). Comparison of weight-loss diets with different compositions of fat, protein, and carbohydrates. *New England Journal of Medicine*, 360: 859-873.
12. Dansinger, M.L., Gleason, J.A., Griffith, J.A., Selker, H.P. Schaefer, E.J. (2005). Comparison of the Atkins, Ornish, Weight Watchers, and Zone Diets for Weight Loss and Heart Disease Risk Reduction: A Randomized Trial. *JAMA*, 293(1):43-53. doi:10.1001/jama.293.1.43.
13. Befort, C.A., Stewart, E.E., Smith, B.K., Gibson, C.A., Sullivan, D.K. and Donnelly, J.E.(2008). Weight maintenance, behaviors and barriers among previous participants of a university-based weight control program. *International Journal of Obesity*, 32, 519–526; doi:10.1038/sj.ijo.0803769.
14. Klem, M. L., Wing, R. R., Lang, W., McGuire, M. T. and Hill, J. O. (2000). Does Weight Loss Maintenance Become Easier Over Time? *Obesity Research*, 8:438–444. doi:10.1038/oby.2000.54.
15. Dr Marsha Marcus of the Western Psychiatric Institute and Clinic in Pittsburgh 102

16. Zhang, X., Qi, Q., Zhang, C., Smith, SR., Hu, FB., Sacks, FM. (2012). FTO Genotype and 2-Year Change in Body Composition and Fat Distribution in Response to Weight-Loss Diets The POUNDS LOST Trial—Diabetes.
17. Qi, Q., Bray, G.A., Smith, S.R., Hu, F.B., Sacks, F.M. and Qi, L. (2011). Insulin Receptor Substrate 1 Gene Variation Modifies Insulin Resistance Response to Weight-Loss Diets in a 2-Year Randomized Trial. The Preventing Overweight Using Novel Dietary Strategies (POUNDS LOST) Trial Circulation.; 124: 563-571 . doi: 10.1161/CIRCULATIONAHA.111.025767.
18. Schick,S.M., Wing, R.R, Klem, M.L., McGuire, M.T., Hill, J.O. & Seagle, H.M. (1998). Persons successful at long-term weight loss and maintenance continue to consume a low calorie, low fat diet. *Journal of the American Dietetic Association*, 98, 408-413.
19. Avenell, A. (2004). Systematic review of the long-term effects and economic consequences of treatments for obesity and implications for health improvement'. *Health Technology Assessment*, 8 (21), 1-182.
20. Dulloo, A.G.(2005) Suppressed thermogenesis as a cause for resistance to slimming and obesity rebound: adaptation or illusion? *Int J Obes*, 31: 201–203.
21. Chaston, T.B., Dixon J.B. and O'Brien, P.E. (2007). Changes in fat-free mass during significant weight loss: a systematic review. *Int J Obes*, 31(5):743-50.
22. van Itallie, T. (1980). Dietary application to the treatment of obesity. In A. Stunkard (ed). *Obesity*. Philadelphia. WB Sanders, 249-261.
23. Clark, M.J. & Slavin, J.L.(2013). The Effect of Fiber on Satiety and Food Intake: A Systematic Review. *Journal of the American College of Nutrition*, 32, 3, 200-211. DOI: 10.1080/07315724.2013. 791194.

Chapter 16: How the New Science in Exercise Can Boost Your Weight Loss

1. Jensen, M.D., Ryan, D.H., Apovian, C.M., Ard J.D., Comuzzie, A.G., Donato, K.A., Hu, F.B., Hubbard V.S, Jakicic, J.M., Kushner, R.F, Loria C, Millen, BE, Nonas, C.A, Pi-Sunyer F.X., Stevens, J., Stevens V.J, Wadden, T.A., Wolfe, B.M. and Yanovski, S.Z. (2013) AHA/ACC/TOS guideline for the management of overweight and obesity in adults: a report of the American College of Cardiology/American Heart Association Task Force on Practice Guidelines and The Obesity Society. *Circulation*. 2013;00:000–000
2. http://www.nwcr.ws/research/
3. Shaw, K.A, Gennat, H.C., O'Rourke P. & Del Mar, C. (2006). Exercise for overweight or obesity. Cochrane Library
4. Curioni, C.C.& Lourenco, P.M. (2005). Long-term weight loss after diet and exercise: a systematic review. *International Journal of Obesity*, 29:1168-74.
5. Dumbrowski, S.U., Knittle, K., Avenell, A., Araújo-Soares, V. & Sniehotta, F.F. (2014). Long term maintenance of weight loss with non-surgical interventions in obese adults: systematic review and meta analyses of randomised controlled trials. *British Medical Journal*, 348 doi: http://dx.doi.org/10.1136/bmj.g2646, 348:g2646
6. Villanova, N., Pasqui1, F., Burzacchini1, S., Forlani, G., Manini, R., Suppini, A., Melchionda, N. and Marchesini, G. (2006). A physical activity program to reinforce weight maintenance following a behavior program in overweight/obese subjects. *International Journal of Obesity*, 30, 697–703. doi:10.1038/sj.ijo.0803185.
7. Delany, J.P., Kelley D.E., Hames, K.C., Jakicic, J.M., Goodpaster, B.H. (2014). Effect of physical activity on weight loss, energy expenditure, and energy intake during diet induced weight loss. *Obesity* (Silver Spring): 22: 363-370.

8. 8.Duncan, L.R., Hall, C.R.,Wilson, P.M. & Rodgers, W.M. (2012). The use of a mental imagery intervention to enhance integrated regulation for exercise among women commencing an exercise program. *Motivation and Emotion*, 36 (4), 452-464.
9. Melanson, E.L. MacLean, P.S. and Hill, J.O. (2009). Exercise improves fat metabolism in muscle but does not increase 24-h fat oxidation. *Exerc Sport Sci Rev*, 37(2): 93–101. doi:10.1097/JES.0b013e31819c2f0b
10. Weiss, E.P., Racette, S.B., Villareal, D.T., Fontana, L., Steger-May, K. Schechtman, K.B., Klein, S., Ehsani, A.A., Holloszy, J.O. (2007). Lower extremity muscle size and strength and aerobic capacity decrease with caloric restriction but not with exercise-induced weight loss. *Journal of Applied Physiology*, 102(2), 634-640 DOI: 10.1152/japplphysiol.00853.2006
11. Desprésa, J. and Lamarche, B. (1993). Effects of Diet and Physical Activity on Adiposity and Body Fat Distribution: Implications for the Prevention of Cardiovascular Disease. *Nutrition Research Reviews*, 6, pp 137-159. doi:10.1079/NRR19930010.
12. Genton, L., Melzer, K. & Pichard, C. (2010). Energy and macronutrient requirements for physical fitness in exercising subjects. *Clin Nutr.*, 29(4): 413–423. doi:10.1016/j.clnu.2010.02.002.
13. Simpson, K.A. & Singh, M.A.(2008). Effects of exercise on adiponectin: a systematic review. *Obesity* (Silver Spring); 16(2): 241-256.
14. King, N.A., Burley, V.J. & Blundell, J.E. (1994). Exercise-induced suppression of appetite: effects on food intake and implications for energy balance. *Eur J Clin Nutr*; 48: 715–724.
15. Holmstrup, M. E., Fairchild, T. J., Keslacy, S., Weinstock, R. S. and Kanaley, J. A. (2013), Satiety, but not total PYY, is increased with continuous and intermittent exercise. *Obesity*, 21: 2014–2020. doi:10.1002/oby.20335.

16. Villarroya, F. (2012). Irisin: turn up the heat. *Cell Metabolism*, 15 (3), 277-278. doi/org/10.1016/j.cmet.2012.02.010.
17. Davis, C.L.; Tomporowski, P.D., McDowell, J. E.; Austin, B.P.; Miller, P. H.; Yanasak, N.E.; Allison, J, D.; Naglieri, J. A. (2011). Exercise improves executive function and achievement and alters brain activation in overweight children: A randomized, controlled trial. *Health Psychology*, 30(1), 91-98. http://dx.doi.org/10.1037/a0021766
18. calorie calculation
19. Shaw. K.A, Gennat, H.C., O'Rourke, P., Del Mar, C. (2006). Exercise for overweight or obesity. Cochrane Library.
20. http://www.cdc.gov/physicalactivity/basics/pa-health/
21. Salmon, P. (2001). Effects of physical exercise on anxiety, depression, and sensitivity to stress: a unifying theory. *Clin Psychol Rev.*, 21(1):33-61.
22. Nieman, D.C. and Pedersen, B.K. (1999). Exercise and Immune Function. Recent Developments. *Sports Medicine*, 27, 2, 73-80.
23. Yang, P., Ho, K., Chen, H., Chien, M (2012). Exercise Training improves sleep quality in middle aged and older adults with sleep problems. a systematic review. *Journal of Physiotherapy,* 58, 3, 157-163. doi. 10.1016518369553C12. 70106-6.
24. Spence, J. C., McGannon, K. R., & Poon, P. (2005). The effect of exercise on global self-esteem: A quantitative review. *Journal of Sport & Exercise Psychology*, 27(3), 311-334.
25. Author (2013). The Association between midlife cardiorespiratory fitness levels and later-life dementia: a cohort study. *Annals of Internal Medicine*, 158, 162.
26. Labban, J. D., & Etnier, J. L. (2011). Effects of acute exercise on long-term memory. *Research Quarterly for Exercise and Sport,* 82(4), 712-21.

Retrieved from http://search.proquest.com/docview/912383838?accountid=166958.

27. Hötting, K., & Röder, B. (2013). Beneficial effects of physical exercise on neuroplasticity and cognition. *Neuroscience and Biobehavioral Reviews*, 37(9), 2243-2257. doi:http://dx.doi.org/10.1016/j.neubiorev.2013.04.005.
28. Bryner, R.W., Ullrich, I.H., Sauers, J., Donley.D., Hornsby, G., Kolar, M. and Yeater, R. (1999). Effects of Resistance vs. Aerobic Training Combined With an 800 Calorie Liquid Diet on Lean Body Mass and Resting Metabolic Rate. *Journal of the American College of Nutrition*, 18, (2), 115-121 .DOI:10.1080/07315724.1999.10718838.
29. Willis, L.H., Slentz, C.A., Bateman, L.A., Shields, T., Piner, L.W., Bales, C.W., Houmard, J.A., Kraus, W.E. (2012). Effects of aerobic and/or resistance training on body mass and fat mass in overweight or obese adults. *Journal of Applied Physiology*, 113, 12, 1831-1837 DOI: 10.1152/japplphysiol. 01370.2011.
30. Herring, L. Y., Wagstaff, C. and Scott, A. (2014), The efficacy of 12weeks supervised exercise in obesity management. *Clinical Obesity*, 4: 220–227. doi: 10.1111/cob.12063
31. Carey, D.G. (2009). Quantifying Differences in the "Fat Burning" Zone and the Aerobic Zone: Implications For Training. *Journal of Strength & Conditioning Research*, 23(7), 2090-2095. doi: 10.1519/JSC.0b013e3181bac5c5.
32. 31.http://www.heart.org/HEARTORG/GettingHealthy/PhysicalActivity/FitnessBasics/Target-Heart-Rates_ UCM_434341_Article.jsp.
33. https://www.nhlbi.nih.gov/health/health-topics/topics/phys/recommend
34. obesity management guidelines for exercise
35. www.csep.ca/CMFIles/Guidelines/CSEP_PAGuidelines_adults_en.pdf
36. Australia, The National Physical Activity Guidelines (2014).

37. Jakicic, J.M., Marcus, B.H., Gallagher, K.I., Napolitano, M. and Lang, W. (2003). Effect of Exercise Duration and Intensity on Weight Loss in Overweight, Sedentary Women: A Randomized Trial. *JAMA*, 290(10):1323-1330. doi:10.1001/jama.290.10.1323
38. Schmidt, W., Anderson, K., Graff, M.., Strutz V. (2015.). The effect of high-intensity circuit training on physical fitness. *The Journal of Sports Medicine and Physical Fitness.*
39. Alizadeh, Z., Kordi, R., Rostami, M., Mansournia, M. A., Hosseinzadeh-Attar, S. M. J., & Fallah, J. (2013). Comparison Between the Effects of Continuous and Intermittent Aerobic Exercise on Weight Loss and Body Fat Percentage in Overweight and Obese Women: A Randomized Controlled Trial. *International Journal of Preventive Medicine*, 4(8), 881–888.
40. Trapp, E.G. Chisholm, D.J., Freund, J. and Boutcher, S.H. (2008). The effects of high-intensity intermittent exercise training on fat loss and fasting insulin levels of young women. *International Journal of Obesity*, 32, 684–691; doi:10.1038/sj.ijo.0803781.
41. Boutcher, S.H.(2011). High-Intensity Intermittent Exercise and Fat Loss. *J Obes*.868305. doi: 10.1155/2011/868305
42. Paoli, A., Moro, T., Marcolin, G., Neri, M., Bianco, A,. Palma, A. and Grimaldi, K. (2012). High-Intensity Interval Resistance Training (HIRT) influences resting energy expenditure and respiratory ratio in non-dieting individuals. *J Translational Med*, 10: 237. doi: 10.1186/1479-5876-10-237
43. Keating, S.E., Machan, E.A., O'Connor, H.T., Gerofi, J.A. Sainsbury, A., Caterson, I.D. and Johnson, N.A. (2014). Continuous Exercise but Not High Intensity Interval Training Improves Fat Distribution in Overweight Adults. *Journal of Obesity*, Article ID 834865. http://dx.doi.org/10.1155/2014/834865.
44. Willcutts, K.F., Wilcox, A.R., Grunewald, K.K.(1988). Energy metabolism during exercise at different time intervals following a meal. *Int J Sports Med*. 9(3):240-3.

45. 44.Gonzalez, J.T., Veasey, R.C., Rumbold, P.L.S. and Stevenson, E.J. (2013). Breakfast and exercise contingently affect postprandial metabolism and energy balance in physically active males. *British Journal of Nutrition*, 1. DOI: 10.1017/S0007114512005582.
46. Maraki, M., Tsofliou, F., Pitsiladis, Y. P., Malkova, D., Mutrie, N., & Higgins, S. (2005). Acute effects of a single exercise class on appetite, energy intake and mood. Is there a time of day effect? *Appetite*, *45*(3), 272-278.
47. Tipton, K.D., Rasmussen, B.B., Miller,S.L. et al. (2001). Timing of amino acid-carbohydrate ingestion alters anabolic response of muscle to resistance exercise. *Am. J. Physiol. Endocrinol. Metab.* 281:E197–E206.
48. Shrier, I. (2005). When and whom to stretch? Gauging the benefits and drawbacks for individual patients. *Phys Sportsmed,* 33(3), 22-26.
49. White, M.P., Pahl, S., Katherine J. Ashbullby K.J., Burton , F. and Depledge, M.H.(2015). The Effects of Exercising in Different Natural Environments on Psycho-Physiological Outcomes in Post-Menopausal Women: A Simulation Study. Int. J. Environ. Res. *Public Health*, 12(9), 11929-11953; doi:10.3390/ijerph120911929.
50. 49.Abraham, C. and Sheeran, P. (2004). Deciding to exercise: The role of anticipated regret. *British Journal of Health Psychology,* 9: 269–278. doi:10.1348/135910704773891096
51. Terbizan, D. J., Dolezal, B. A., & Albano, C. (2002). Validity of seven commercially available heart rate monitors. *Measurement in Physical Education and Exercise Science*, *6*(4), 243-247.
52. Dunstan, D.W., Howard, B., Healy, G.N., Owen, N. (2012). Too much sitting—A health hazard. *Diabetes Research and Clinical Practice*, 97(3), 368–376 DOI: http://dx.doi.org/10.1016/j.diabres.2012.05.020

53. Miller, J.M. (2007). The energy expenditure of using a "walk-and-work" desk for office workers with obesity," *British Journal of Sports Medicine*, 41(9), 558-561. J. A. Levine
54. Rudolph,D.L.&McAuley,E.(1998).Cortisolandaffective responses to exercise. *Journal of Sports Sciences*, 16 (2), 121-128. DOI:10.1080/026404198366830.

Appendix 1: Tracking Your Progress

1. Nackers, L. M., Ross, K. M., & Perri, M. G. (2010). The association between rate of initial weight loss and long-term success in obesity treatment: Does slow and steady win the race? *International Journal of Behavioral Medicine*, 17(3), 161-7. Retrieved from http://search.proquest.com/docview/745603466?accountid=166958
2. Slomski, A., M.A. (2014). No difference in weight regain from fast or slow diet. *JAMA, 312*(24), 2609. Retrieved from http://search.proquest.com/docview/1644105565?accountid=166958
3. Elfhag, K. and Rössner, S. (2005). Who succeeds in maintaining weight loss? A conceptual review of factors associated with weight loss maintenance and weight regain. *Obesity Reviews*, 6, (1) 67–85.
4. Faryle, N. & Jingzhen,Y. (2007). Goal setting frequency and the use of behavioral strategies related to diet and physical activity. *Health Education Research*, 22(4): 532-8.
5. Rosenbaum, M., Kissileff, H.R., Mayer, L.E., Hirsch, J., Leibel, R.L.(2010). Energy intake in weight-reduced humans. *Brain Research*, 1350: 95-102.
6. Kaplan, L.M., Seeley, R.J. and Harris, J.L. (2012). Myths associated with obesity and bariatric surgery. *Bariatric Times*, 9(4):12–13.
7. Lutes, L.D., Winett, R.A, Barger, S.D, et al. 2008). Small changes in nutrition and physical activity promote weight loss and maintenance: 3-month evidence

from the ASPIRE randomized trial. *Ann Behavioral Medicine*, 35:351–7.
8. 8.Wadden, T.A., Foster G.D., Letizia, K.A. (1994) One-year behavioral treatment of obesity: comparison of moderate and severe caloric restriction and the effects of weight maintenance therapy. *J Consult Clin Psychol*, 62:165–71
9. Maclean, P.S., Bergouignan, A., Cornier, M.A., Jackman M.R. (2011). Biology's response to dieting: the impetus for weight regain. *American Journal of Physiol Regul Integre Comp Physiology*, 301: R581-R600.
10. MacLean, P.S., Higgins, J.A., Jackman, M.R., et al. (2006) Peripheral metabolic responses to prolonged weight reduction that promote rapid, efficient regain in obesity-prone rats. *American Journal Physiological Regulations Integret Comp Physiology,* 290: R1577-R1588
11. Elfhag, K.and Rössner, S. (2005). Who succeeds in maintaining weight loss? A conceptual review of factors associated with weight loss maintenance and weight regain. *Obesity Reviews*, 6, (1), 67–85.
12. Guyenet, S.J. & Schwartz, M.W. (2012). Clinical review: regulation of food intake, energy balance, and body fat mass: implications for the pathogenesis and treatment of obesity. *Journal of Clinical and Endocrinological Metabolism*, 97, 745–55.
13. Rosenbaum, M., Kissileff, H.R., Mayer, L.E., Hirsch, J., Leibel, R.L.(2010). Energy intake in weight-reduced humans. *Brain Research*, 1350: 95-102.

Appendix 2: Monitor Your Behaviours

1. Klem, M.L., Wing, R.R., Lang, W., McGuire, M.T. and Hill, J.O. (2000). Does Weight Loss Maintenance Become Easier Over Time? *Obesity Research*, 8:438–444.
2. Kayman, S., Bruvold, W. and Stern, J.S.(1990). Maintenance and relapse after weight loss in women:

behavioral aspects. *American Journal of Clinical Nutrition*, 52 (5), 800-807.

Appendix 3: Alcohol and Your Weight

1. Hagan, M. M., Shuman, E. S., Oswald, K. D., Corcoran, K. J., & al, e. (2002). Incidence of chaotic eating behaviors in binge-eating disorder: Contributing factors. *Behavioral Medicine*, 28(3), 99-105. Retrieved from http://search.proquest.com/docview/195223698?accountid=166958
2. Chapman, C. D., Benedict, C., Brooks, S. J., & Schiöth, H.B. (2012). Lifestyle determinants of the drive to eat: A meta-analysis. The American Journal of Clinical Nutrition, 96(3), 492-497. doi:http://dx.doi.org/10.3945/ajcn.112.039750
3. Calorieking.com
4. Mulhall, B. P., Ong, J. P. and Younossi, Z. M. (2002). Non-alcoholic fatty liver disease: An overview. *Journal of Gastroenterology and Hepatology*, 17:1136–1143. doi:10.1046/j.1440-1746.2002.02881x
5. World Health Organization. AUDIT.

Made in United States
Orlando, FL
05 November 2026

90230631R00199